Fast Facts for the CRITICAL CARE NURSE: Critical Care Nursing in a Nutshell (*Landrum*)

Fast Facts for the TRAVEL NURSE: Travel Nursing in a Nutshell (*Landrum*)

Fast Facts for the SCHOOL NURSE: School Nursing in a Nutshell, Second Edition (*Loschiavo*)

Fast Facts for MANAGING PATIENTS WITH A PSYCHIATRIC DISORDER: What RNs, NPs, and New Psych Nurses Need to Know (*Marshall*)

Fast Facts About CURRICULUM DEVELOPMENT IN NURSING: How to Develop and Evaluate Educational Programs in a Nutshell, Second Edition (*McCoy, Anema*)

Fast Facts About NEUROCRITICAL CARE: A Quick Reference for the Advanced Practice Provider (*McLaughlin*)

Fast Facts for DEMENTIA CARE: What Nurses Need to Know in a Nutshell (*Miller*)

Fast Facts for HEALTH PROMOTION IN NURSING: Promoting Wellness in a Nutshell (*Miller*)

Fast Facts for STROKE CARE NURSING: An Expert Care Guide, Second Edition (*Morrison*)

Fast Facts for the MEDICAL OFFICE NURSE: What You Really Need to Know in a Nutshell (*Richmeier*)

Fast Facts for the PEDIATRIC NURSE: An Orientation Guide in a Nutshell (*Rupert, Young*)

Fast Facts About the GYNECOLOGICAL EXAM: A Professional Guide for NPs, PAs, and Midwives, Second Edition (*Secor, Fantasia*)

Fast Facts for the STUDENT NURSE: Nursing Student Success in a Nutshell (*Stabler-Haas*)

Fast Facts for CAREER SUCCESS IN NURSING: Making the Most of Mentoring in a Nutshell (*Vance*)

Fast Facts for the TRIAGE NURSE: An Orientation and Care Guide in a Nutshell (*Visser, Montejano, Grossman*)

Fast Facts for DEVELOPING A NURSING ACADEMIC PORTFOLIO: What You Really Need to Know in a Nutshell (*Wittmann-Price*)

Fast Facts for the HOSPICE NURSE: A Concise Guide to End-of-Life Care (*Wright*)

Fast Facts for the CLASSROOM NURSING INSTRUCTOR: Classroom Teaching in a Nutshell (*Yoder-Wise, Kowalski*)

Forthcoming FAST FACTS Books

Fact Facts in HEALTH INFORMATICS (*Hardy*)

Fact Facts About NURSE ANESTHESIA (*Hickman*)

Fast Facts for the CARDIAC SURGERY NURSE, Third Edition (*Hodge*)

Fast Facts for the CRITICAL CARE NURSE: Critical Care Nursing, Second Edition (*Landrum*)

Fast Facts for the SCHOOL NURSE, Third Edition (*Loschiavo*)

Fast Facts on How to Conduct, Understand, and Maybe Even Love RESEARCH! For Nurses and Other Healthcare Providers (*Marshall*)

Fast Facts About SUBSTANCE ABUSE DISORDERS: What Every Nurse, APRN, and PA Needs to Know (*Marshall, Spencer*)

Fast Facts for the CATH LAB NURSE (*McCulloch*)

Fast Facts About FORENSIC NURSING: What You Need to Know (*Scannell*)

Fast Facts About RELIGION IN NURSING: Implications for Patient Care (*Taylor*)

Fast Facts for the TRIAGE NURSE: An Orientation and Care Guide, Second Edition (*Visser*)

Visit www.springerpub.com to order.

FAST FACTS About
NEUROCRITICAL CARE

Diane McLaughlin, DNP, AGACNP-BC, CCRN, is a critical care nurse practitioner who works in the departments of neurosurgery and neurocritical care at MetroHealth Medical Center in Cleveland, Ohio, and in critical care at Mayo Clinic in Jacksonville, Florida. Dr. McLaughlin has worked in critical care for 15 years, first as a nurse and then as a nurse practitioner. She received her master of science in nursing from the University of Florida in 2013 and her doctorate of nursing practice from the University of Florida in 2017. Her research interests include neurosurveillance, sleep in critical care, and advanced practice provider training and education.

Dr. McLaughlin is active within the Society of Critical Care Medicine, serving 3-year appointments to both the Adult Ultrasound Committee and the Advanced Practice Provider Resource Committee. She has also served as faculty for the SCCM Ultrasound Fundamentals Course. Dr. McLaughlin is also active within the Neurocritical Care Society, having served as a reviewer and currently serving on a guideline writing committee. Dr. McLaughlin is also a member of the American Association of Critical Care Nurses and American Association of Nurse Practitioners. She has spoken at multiple local, national, and international conferences on topics in neurocritical care and has published regarding topics in critical care, neurocritical care, and advanced practice provider use in critical care.

FAST FACTS About
NEUROCRITICAL CARE

A Quick Reference for the Advanced Practice Provider

Diane McLaughlin, DNP, AGACNP-BC, CCRN

SPRINGER PUBLISHING COMPANY

Springer Publishing Company, LLC
11 West 42nd Street
New York, NY 10036
www.springerpub.com

Acquisitions Editor: Elizabeth Nieginski
Compositor: Amnet

ISBN: 978-0-8261-8819-9
ebook ISBN: 978-0-8261-8823-6

19 20 21 22 23 / 5 4 3 2 1

The author and the publisher of this Work have made every effort to use sources believed to be reliable to provide information that is accurate and compatible with the standards generally accepted at the time of publication. Because medical science is continually advancing, our knowledge base continues to expand. Therefore, as new information becomes available, changes in procedures become necessary. We recommend that the reader always consult current research and specific institutional policies before performing any clinical procedure. The author and publisher shall not be liable for any special, consequential, or exemplary damages resulting, in whole or in part, from the readers' use of, or reliance on, the information contained in this book. The publisher has no responsibility for the persistence or accuracy of URLs for external or third-party Internet websites referred to in this publication and does not guarantee that any content on such websites is, or will remain, accurate or appropriate.

Library of Congress Cataloging-in-Publication Data
Names: McLaughlin, Diane (Diane C.), author.
Title: Fast facts about neurocritical care : a quick reference for the advanced practice provider / Diane McLaughlin.
Description: New York, NY : Springer Publishing Company, LLC, [2019] |
  Series: Fast facts | Includes bibliographical references and index.
Identifiers: LCCN 2018027705 (print) | LCCN 2018028118 (ebook) | ISBN 9780826188236 |
  ISBN 9780826188199 | ISBN 9780826188236 (e-book)
Subjects: | MESH: Nervous System Diseases—nursing | Critical Care Nursing—methods |
  Advanced Practice Nursing—methods | Handbooks
Classification: LCC RC86.8 (ebook) | LCC RC86.8 (print) | NLM WY 49 | DDC
  616.02/8—dc23
LC record available at https://lccn.loc.gov/2018027705

Contact us to receive discount rates on bulk purchases.
We can also customize our books to meet your needs.
For more information, please contact sales@springerpub.com

Publisher's Note: New and used products purchased from third-party sellers are not guaranteed for quality, authenticity, or access to any included digital components.

Printed in the United States of America.

*This book is dedicated to Dr. William David Freeman,
who woke up at 4 a.m. on Saturday mornings just to teach me.
His mentorship and encouragement continue
to inspire me to explore the unknown, teach the known, and
always strive to reach higher.*

Contents

Contents

Foreword

If you are an advanced practice provider (APP), you should obtain this book. If you are working in neurology, neurosurgery, or critical care, you *need* this book. As a practicing physician assistant for over 22 years, I have seen a dramatic change in the acceptance of APPs as integral partners in healthcare. The demand on our healthcare system has put an ever-increasing need for our patients and loved ones to rely on an advocate and mediator to care for them. There are very few resources that are specific to neurology critical care and neurosurgery APPs. This book, authored by Diane McLaughlin, meets those expectations.

Starting with the basic neurology exam and then thoroughly walking you through the different types of strokes, trauma, infectious diseases, seizures, and brain death criteria, this practical and commonsense approach is an excellent companion to the care you provide to your patient.

I have had the good fortune of working directly with Dr. McLaughlin at Mayo Clinic since 2013, sharing patients and exchanging ideas. Her vast experience in critical care and expertise in clinical trials and studies places her at the top of her field in patient care and research. I am honored to work with her and care for the critical needs of our patients and their families.

Grace H. Bryan, PA-C
Mayo Clinic Jacksonville Neurosurgery
President, Association of Neurosurgical Physician Assistants

Preface

Welcome to *Fast Facts About Neurocritical Care: A Quick Reference for the Advanced Practice Provider*. This book is a very nonexclusive resource for *anyone* who works in neurocritical care, including physician assistants, nurse practitioners, clinical nurse specialists, and bedside nurses. I would not even be surprised to find it in the hands of a medical student, intern, or resident.

If you are reading this book, then you probably already take care of neurology patients. This also means that you already realize that neurology is a challenging specialty. Lack of knowledge regarding how to perform an adequate neurological examination, how to diagnose specific conditions, and, perhaps most importantly, how to treat them, can be dangerous for both the patient and provider.

This book will not tell a story. This book will not provide in-depth anatomy, pathophysiology, or pharmacology. Instead, this book will give you exactly what the title portrays—a quick reference book to give you "fast facts" about commonly seen neurological conditions in the adult critical care setting. You will also receive some pearls of wisdom, some useful tables, and even some scoring guides to help you assess your patients and classify their pathology. This book is best suited for a work bag or office desk to reference when you forget whether seizure prophylaxis is indicated, cannot find your stroke scale booklet, or are unsure which tests you should order during a meningitis workup. I hope it serves you well and that you use it often.

Diane McLaughlin

I

The Neuro Exam

1

The Neurological Examination

The goal of the neurological examination is to identify the area of the brain that is compromised. The use of serial examinations helps identify improvement or worsening of the injury to ensure early intervention. These serial checks are commonly referred to as "neuro checks." The frequency of neuro checks is often based upon the patient's potential for deterioration due to the sequela of the disease process. The exam itself may be focused dependent upon the patient's status, as you will see from the coming chapters. The following chapters will detail and explain what is involved in a neuro check.

In this chapter, you will learn how to:

- Identify components of a neuro check.
- Avoid common pitfalls of the neurological examination.
- Review common exam features based upon the area of injury (localization).

COMPONENTS OF A NEURO CHECK

The neuro check consists of many components. A thorough neuro check includes level of consciousness (LOC), Glasgow Coma Scale (GCS), speech, orientation, cranial nerve (CN) examination, sensation, motor strength, reflexes, and maybe assessment of gait.

Level of Consciousness

LOC broadly refers to the patient's wakefulness and ability to interact with the environment around him or her. In critical care, we typically utilize five different terms to describe LOC.

- **Alert:** This is the typical LOC of awake human beings. The patient is awake and interactive.
- **Lethargic:** The patient is drowsy but can be aroused with verbal or physical stimuli, but the patient returns to drowsiness when stimuli are removed.
- **Obtunded:** This patient is lethargic but requires increased stimuli to promote wakefulness; however, the patient is less interactive with the environment with decreased response to stimulation.
- **Stupor:** The patient only arouses to vigorous and repeated stimuli. If stimulation is not introduced, the patient is in an unresponsive state without interaction with his or her surrounding environment.
- **Coma:** The patient is unable to be aroused, is unresponsive, and does not interact with his or her environment.

Fast Facts

If you are unsure of the proper term to categorize LOC, describe the patient response to stimuli.

Glasgow Coma Scale

GCS is a commonly used scale to objectively measure LOC (Table 1.1). The lowest score a patient can receive is 3 and the highest is 15. GCS score less than 8 is associated with a comatose state. The total GCS score is based upon the best score from each category.

Common Pitfalls

- Common pitfalls of assessment of GCS eye response: Sleeping patients who easily awaken should still receive a score of 4. If application of noxious stimuli is required to assess for eye opening, nail bed pressure is often more effective than trapezius squeeze or sternal rub, which is likely to elicit grimacing.
- Common pitfalls of assessment of GCS verbal response: Inappropriate words (3) should be scored when a patient has random words or shouts but is unable to participate in conversation. Patients receive a score of 4 (confusion) when they are able to respond

Table 1.1

Glasgow Coma Scale		
Eye Response	Verbal Response	Motor Response
1—No eye opening	1—No verbal response	1—No motor response
2—Eye opening to noxious stimuli	2—Incomprehensible sounds	2—Extension to noxious stimuli
3—Eye opening to speech	3—Inappropriate words	3—Abnormal flexion to noxious stimuli
4—Spontaneous eye opening	4—Confused	4—Withdrawal to noxious stimuli
	5—Oriented	5—Localizes to noxious stimuli
		6—Follows commands

coherently, however, with confusion or disorientation. Patients receive a score of 2 (incomprehensible sounds) for general moaning without an attempt at words or an attempt at speech that is not understandable.

■ Common pitfalls of assessment of GCS motor response: Confusion often exists between extension, flexion, and withdrawal response. Extension refers to external shoulder rotation with extension of the wrist. Conversely, with flexion, the shoulder rotates internally with flexion of the wrist. Withdrawal response refers to a patient's withdrawal to noxious stimuli when he or she pulls his or her extremity away from nail bed pressure.

Speech/Language

Speech can be easily assessed during routine neurological examination and does not need specific tests to make observations. The examiner should note the following:

■ Quality of speech: Hoarse, whispery, slurred, or garbled
■ Fluency: Fluent/fluid, cluttering/tachyphrasia (rapid and erratic), stuttering, slow or halting speech
■ Presence of other language disorders

Orientation

The assessment of orientation has many purposes. First, the examiner is able to observe the patient's attentiveness and ability to comprehend. Examiners also are able to assess the patient's speech and language patterns. Orientation questions (name, time/date, location) test the patient's short- and long-term memory.

Cranial Nerve Examination

The CNs originate primarily from the brainstem, with the exception of CN I and II, which originate from the cerebrum (Figure 1.1; Table 1.2).

- CN I—The olfactory nerve
  - The olfactory nerve can be tested by having the patient occlude each nostril, close his or her eyes, and identify scents (soap, vanilla, coffee, etc.).
  - Hyposmia (diminished sense of smell) can occur for many reasons. Hyperosmia can occur with Addison's disease. Anosmia is the inability to recognize odors and is most likely to occur with brain injury. Head trauma, such as injury to the occiput, can cause this. Anterior fossa tumors can cause unilateral anosmia. Meningitis or subarachnoid hemorrhage can also cause anosmia.
- CN II—The optic nerve
  - There are multiple tests to evaluate the optic nerve.
    - Funduscopic exam: The primary purpose of the funduscopic examination in this patient population is to evaluate for the presence of papilledema.

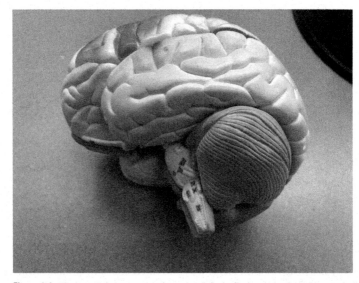

Figure 1.1 The cranial nerves can be seen (labeled) along the brainstem.

Table 1.2

Cranial Nerves

Cranial Nerve	Origin	Motor/Sensory/Both	Function
I: Olfactory	Cerebrum	Sensory	Smell
II: Optic	Cerebrum	Sensory	Visual acuity, visual fields, pupillary reactions, ocular fundi
III: Oculomotor	Midbrain–pontine junction	Motor	Pupillary reactions, extraocular movement
IV: Trochlear	Posterior side of midbrain	Motor	Extraocular movement
V: Trigeminal	Pons	Both	Facial sensation, movements of the jaw, corneal reflexes, voice and speech
VI: Abducens	Pontine–medulla junction	Motor	Extraocular movement
VII: Facial	Pontine–medulla junction	Both	Facial movement, gustation, voice and speech
VIII: Vestibulocochlear	Pontine–medulla junction	Sensory	Hearing and balance
IX: Glossopharyngeal	Medulla oblongata, posterior to the olive	Both	Swallowing, palate elevation, gag reflex, gustation
X: Vagus	Medulla oblongata, posterior to the olive	Both	Swallowing, palate elevation, gag reflex, gustation, voice and speech
XI: Spinal	Medulla oblongata, posterior to the olive	Motor	Shrugging of the shoulders, turning the head
XII: Hypoglossal	Medulla oblongata, anterior to the olive	Motor	Movement and protrusion of the tongue, voice and speech

❑ Visual fields: These can be tested by asking the patient to focus on the examiner's nose (approximately 1–2 feet away) and report how many fingers the examiner is showing in each quadrant, utilizing his or her peripheral vision. This can be done with the patient having both eyes open (binocular) or one eye open at a time (monocular). Specific terminology can help describe defects (Figure 1.2).

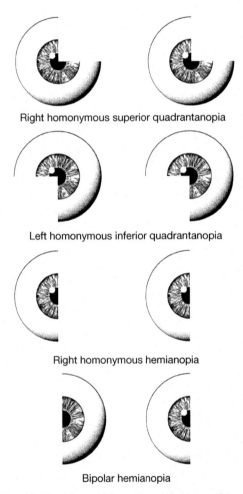

Right homonymous superior quadrantanopia

Left homonymous inferior quadrantanopia

Right homonymous hemianopia

Bipolar hemianopia

Figure 1.2 Visual fields and terminology. The omitted part of the eye signifies the area of vision that is absent.
Illustration: Nicholas McLaughlin.

- ❑ Visual extinction: This can be tested by showing fingers to the patient on both sides at the same time. The patient is then asked to add how many total fingers are being shown.
- ❑ Visual acuity: Each eye is tested separately. Patients who have corrective glasses/contacts should wear them. A Snellen chart is used to determine visual acuity from 20 feet. A quantitative assessment should be recorded for each eye (e.g., 20/20). More likely in the critical care setting, a handheld chart is utilized to test visual acuity. This is held approximately 14 inches from the patient's face and it otherwise is similar to the Snellen chart.
  - ▪ Significance: Each exam has a specific purpose. Visual fields are important and help localize the lesion anteriorly or posteriorly to the optic chiasm. Anterior lesions will cause visual field deficits in one eye, whereas posterior lesions will cause visual field deficits in both eyes. If visual extinction or hemineglect is present, most commonly there is a contralateral parietal lesion; however, this may also be caused by thalamic or frontal lesions.
- ▪ CN II and CN III—The oculomotor nerve
  - ▪ The oculomotor nerve can be tested by pupillary examination. First, bilateral pupils are observed for size, shape, and symmetry. Next, a penlight is directed into one eye at a time and both pupils are checked for direct and consensual response to light as well as rate of response. For patients with sluggish or absent light reflex, accommodation is assessed. This is tested by asking the patient to focus on an object (such as the penlight) and the pupils should constrict when it is moved closer to the patient. Also of note, the pupils have both afferent (sensory—CN II) pathway and efferent (motor—CN III) pathways, which can be evaluated at this time. CN II (afferent pathway) can be tested utilizing the swinging light test. In this test the light is swung from one pupil to the other every 2 to 3 seconds. In a normal test, no change occurs. In an abnormal test, suggestive of an afferent lesion, the pupils will dilate (as opposed to constrict) when the light goes from the normal eye to the affected eye.

Fast Facts

Hippus, or brief oscillations of pupil size, may occur normally in response to light and often improves in the dark. Unilateral hippus could indicate CN III compression or herniation. Pathologic causes of bilateral hippus include seizures, hysteria, and meningitis.

■ Significance: Asymmetric pupils (anisocoria) can have varied significance. One fifth of the general population has slight asymmetry of their pupils. New anisocoria, however, often signifies impending herniation and CN III compression.

Fast Facts

To assist in localizing anisocoria, if the right pupil is greater than the left, this should be reassessed in both dim and bright light. If the asymmetry is more pronounced in dim light, then the sympathetic system in the left eye is disrupted and the right eye attempts to compensate by dilating further. If the asymmetry is more pronounced in bright light, the presence of a parasympathetic lesion in the right eye should be suspected.

■ CN III, CN IV—the trochlear nerve—and CN VI—the abducens nerve
  ■ CNs III, IV, and VI are tested by observing extraocular eye movements (EOMs). This is done by asking the patient to follow your finger or a penlight with just his or her eyes, keeping his or her head still. Assessment patterns are detailed in Figure 1.3. Note palsies and nystagmus (horizontal or vertical).
  ■ Significance: Inability to move the eyes in a particular direction is called a gaze palsy and is often present in central lesions. This is also called a conjugate lesion. If the eyes cannot be voluntarily moved in the confined direction, but do move in that direction with reflex movements, then the lesion is cortical. If the eyes are unable to be moved to the confined direction voluntarily or by reflex, then the lesion is nuclear and resides in the brainstem. There are many possible causes of nystagmus, including drugs, alcohol, and even fatigue. Vertical

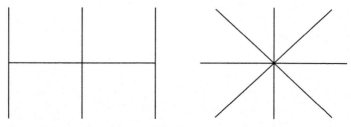

Figure 1.3 Patterns that can be utilized to assess extraocular eye movements.

nystagmus, also called ocular bobbing, is always an abnormal finding and is typical in injury to the pons.

- CN V—the trigeminal nerve
  - Examination of CN V includes both motor and sensory testing. First, to assess motor, ask the patient to bite down. While the patient is doing this, palpate the masseter muscles. Next, the examiner applies gentle resistance against the patient's chin and assesses the patient's ability to open his or her mouth. A jaw jerk reflex should be tested by tapping on the jaw when the mouth is slightly open. To assess sensation, ask the patient to close his or her eyes and state sharp or dull when the patient feels an object (blunt needle vs. cotton wisp) touch his or her face. Corneal testing is also part of the sensory assessment of the trigeminal nerve; however, this is often omitted in the exam of an alert patient.
  - Significance: It is difficult to localize lesions based solely upon CN V assessment findings, as weakness can be caused by upper motor neuron (UMN) pathway lesions, lower motor neuron (LMN) pathway lesions, or even brainstem lesions. The presence of a jaw jerk is more specific and suggests the presence of a UMN lesion.
- CN VII—the facial nerve
  - Observe the patient's face for asymmetry during both conversation and rest. Ask the patient to raise his or her eyebrows, puff his or her cheeks, and show his or her teeth (smile). Assess for both asymmetry and/or any difficulty performing these tasks. Lastly, have the patient close his or her eyes tight and resist eye opening by the examiner. Assess for weakness.
  - Significance: Complete hemiparesis of the face typically suggests a peripheral lesion. If the forehead is spared, the lesion is central and is often associated with stroke. The forehead is innervated by both cerebral hemispheres.
- CN VIII—the vestibulocochlear nerve
  - In the outpatient setting, hearing and conduction testing includes the use of a tuning fork. In the critical care setting, this is not practical. Therefore, assessment of CN VIII is most often limited to the ability of the patient to hear soft speech and assessment of fingers rubbing together bilaterally.
  - Significance: Unilateral hearing loss is suggestive of a peripheral lesion. Bilateral hearing loss is more likely to be centrally located. Most commonly, hearing loss is not due to brain injury, but rather to excessive noise exposure, viral infections, ototoxic medication, or aging.

- CN IX—the glossopharyngeal nerve—and CN X—the vagus nerve
  - Assess CN IX and CN X by noting the patient's vocal quality. Note if the patient has a hoarse or nasal quality to his or her voice. Assess difficulty in patient swallowing. Ask the patient to open his or her mouth and observe the symmetric rise of the soft palate as the patient says "ahh." The gag reflex is also assessed during this portion of the neurological exam; however, it is often omitted in alert patients.
  - Significance: The presence of dysarthria and dysphagia indicates weakness of the muscles innervated by CNs IX and X. Quality of voice may also help localize the lesion. Strained, strangled vocal quality is consistent with a central lesion whereas peripheral lesions are associated with a breathy, nasal, or hoarse voice.
- CN XI—the spinal accessory nerve
  - CN XI is assessed first by observing for muscle weakness. Next, the examiner places both hands on the patient's shoulders and applies gentle resistance while asking the patient to shrug. Then, the examiner has the patient attempt to turn his or her head against resistance. This is repeated on the opposite side. The patient should be able to overcome resistance with equal strength bilaterally.
  - Significance: Central lesions produce ipsilateral sternocleidomastoid (SCM) weakness and contralateral trapezius weakness. Peripheral lesions also produce ipsilateral SCM weakness but also ipsilateral trapezius weakness.
- CN XII—the hypoglossal nerve
  - CN XII is assessed by asking the patient to protrude his or her tongue and move it side to side. Note any deviations from midline or inability to control movements of the tongue.
  - Significance: If a peripheral lesion is present, the tongue deviates toward the side of the lesion. If a central lesion is present, the tongue will deviate away from the lesion.

Fast Facts

The examination of all CNs is not necessary in all patients, particularly in neurocritical care. The examination should be tailored to the patient's history and brain injury.

Fast Facts

Avoid utilizing phrases such as "CNs II–XII grossly intact" unless you actually assess all CNs.

Sensation

The assessment of sensation is subjective and is often limited to these questions: Can the patient feel soft touch and does the patient have paresthesias? In a more detailed exam, the patient will initially be asked about paresthesias (pins and needles) or diminished sensation. This will then be tested symmetrically by asking the patient to close his or her eyes and touching each extremity. The patient will be asked which side you are touching. When you are touching both sides, the patient should be able to identify both; otherwise the patient has extinction. Another test frequently performed to assess sensation is the determination of sharp versus dull.

The pattern of sensory loss can be useful for localization. Cortical lesions are unlikely to affect sensation. The cerebral cortex does have some sensation deficits, such as in parietal lobe damage; these patients may have trouble identifying objects by touch (stereognosis) or recognizing symbols or letters written on their skin (graphesthesia). Lesions in the thalamus have severe contralateral sensation loss with minimal recovery over time. Lesions of the brainstem and spinal cord also have significant effect on sensation and will be detailed more specifically in subsequent chapters.

Motor Exam

There are multiple components to the motor exam, including bulk, tone, strength, and movement.

Bulk is easily observed and refers to muscle volume. Bulk can be categorized utilizing the following terms: atrophy (decreased muscle size), normal, or hypertrophy (increased muscle size).

Tone refers to muscle tension when relaxed or passively moved. Terms used to describe tone include flaccid (no tone), hypotonic (decreased tone), or hypertonic (increased tone). Spastic refers to patients who have an increase in muscle tension when a muscle is lengthened, whereas rigidity refers to a steady state of increased muscle tension.

Hemiplegia is complete *paralysis* of one side. Hemiparesis is *weakness* of one side.

Strength is extremely important to note in the neurological assessment of a patient with brain injury. Muscles typically included in testing consist of the deltoids, biceps, triceps, forearm extensors, forearm flexors and hand muscles, iliopsoas muscles, medial thigh adductors, gluteus maximus and minimus, quadriceps, hamstrings, muscles in the anterior and posterior compartments of the lower leg, and extensor hallucis longus muscle. Strength is graded on a scale of 0 to 5 (Table 1.3). Loss of muscle strength can be categorized as complete or incomplete and may affect one side of the body or all extremities.

Pronator Drift

Perhaps the most important test for UMN weakness is the assessment of pronator drift. For this test, the patients are asked to raise both arms straight out, palms up, and close their eyes. The examiner will ask them to hold their arms there for approximately 10 seconds. For a patient who has UMN weakness, the affected arm will pronate.

A patient faking weakness will often drop his or her arm without pronating it.

Table 1.3

Grades to Describe Muscle Strength

0—No movement

1—Muscle contraction

2—Active movement, not against gravity

3—Antigravity movement

4—Antigravity movement and movement against resistance

5—Normal strength

Table 1.4

DTR Scoring

Score	Description
5+	Sustained clonus
4+	Very brisk, hyperreflexive, with clonus
3+	Brisker or more reflexive than normal
2+	Normal
1+	Low normal, diminished
0	No response

DTR, deep tendon reflexes.

Reflexes

A reflex hammer is utilized to elicit deep tendon reflexes in all extremities. In order to help the patient remain in a relaxed state, it may be useful to ask the patient to clench his or her teeth or interlace fingers and pull apart. The scoring in Table 1.4 should be utilized to describe elicited reflexes.

With the patient relaxed, assess the following reflexes. Compare all reflexes bilaterally.

- Biceps and brachioradialis (C5/C6 nerve roots): Elicited by placing your thumb on the biceps tendon and striking it with the reflex hammer. The brachioradialis reflex is elicited by striking the tendon directly approximately 3 inches above the wrist. The wrist should supinate.
- Triceps (C6/C7 nerve roots): Elicited by directly striking the triceps tendon with reflex hammer while supporting the patient's arm.
- Knee jerk (L3/L4 nerve roots): Elicited by directly striking the quadriceps tendon.
- Ankle (S1 nerve root): Elicited by holding relaxed foot and directly striking the Achilles tendon.

Fast Facts

Cerebellar injury may result in pendular reflexes. Though these reflexes are not brisk, patients with injury to the cerebellum may have a knee jerk that swings back and forth multiple times, whereas a normal response typically has one swing forward and back.

Pathologic Reflexes

- Plantar reflex: Tested by running the opposite end of the reflex hammer along the lateral foot from heel to toe. This is often performed incorrectly by providers who instead run the hammer along the medial aspect of the foot. A normal response would be flexion or no response. Extension, characterized by an upgoing big toe, is a positive Babinski sign.

- Hoffmann response: Elicited by holding the patient's finger between the examiner's thumb and index finger. The examiner's thumb is then deflected downward over the patient's fingernail until the nails "click." No response is normal. A positive Hoffmann sign is seen when flexion of the patient's other fingers occurs after the "click."

- Clonus: Should be tested if any of the patient's reflexes were hyperactive. Hold the patient's leg and ask the patient to relax his or her ankle. The examiner sharply dorsiflexes the patient's foot and holds it in the dorsiflexed position. No response is normal. The patient has clonus if you feel pulsations once the foot is dorsiflexed.

Bibliography

Biller, J., Gruener, G., & Brazis, P. (2011). *DeMyer's the neurologic examination: A programmed text* (6th ed.). New York, NY: McGraw-Hill Medical.

Fuller, G. (2013). *Neurological examination made easy* (5th ed.). Edinburgh, Scotland: Churchill Livingstone/Elsevier.

Lewis, S. L. (2004). *Field guide to the neurologic examination*. Philadelphia, PA: Lippincott Williams & Wilkins.

2

Neurological Examination of a Patient With Stroke

As stated in the previous chapter, the goal of the neurological examination is to identify the area of the brain that is compromised. The National Institute of Health Stroke Scale (NIHSS) is a specific stroke scale commonly used to quantify the assessment of patients with stroke. Providers who do not commonly perform the NIHSS may have trouble scoring patients. This chapter is meant to aid in the scoring of difficult-to-assess patients.

In this chapter, you will learn how to:

- Demonstrate consistent assessment of stroke patients utilizing NIHSS.
- Verbalize understanding of NIHSS in terms of treatment.
- Discuss stroke scale score and its correlation with degree of stroke.

NATIONAL INSTITUTE OF HEALTH STROKE SCALE

Similar to how use of the Glasgow Coma Scale (GCS) allows standardized assessment between providers, the NIHSS is used to quantify the assessment of patients with stroke. The highest NIHSS score possible is 42. This is based upon scoring in 11 items, including level of consciousness (LOC), best gaze, visual field testing, facial paresis,

Table 2.1

The National Institute of Health Stroke Scale Score Is Used to Classify Stroke Severity

0 = No stroke

1–4 = Minor stroke

5–15 = Moderate stroke

16–20 = Moderate/severe stroke

21–42 = Severe stroke

arm and leg motor function, limb ataxia, sensory, best language, dysarthria, and extinction/inattention. The total score the patient receives is associated with the degree of stroke (Table 2.1).

Higher scores are associated with more severe stroke and correlate with infarction size. NIHSS scores within the first 48 hours following stroke also correlate with clinical outcomes at 3 months and 1 year. NIHSS scores of less than 4 are associated with favorable functional outcomes.

Fast Facts

Administration of tissue plasminogen activator (tPA) in patients with an NIHSS score greater than 22 correlates with a higher risk of hemorrhagic conversion.

EXAMINATION

Fast Facts

Record exactly what the patient does. Patients do not get credit for what they have done previously or what you believe they are able to do.

Level of Consciousness

- Overall LOC
  - Escalate level of stimulation until response is achieved: Start with verbal stimulation and then physical, lastly escalating to noxious stimuli.

- 1a LOC scoring
  - ❏ 0 = Alert, keenly responsive
  - ❏ 1 = Not alert but arousable by minor stimulation
  - ❏ 2 = Not alert, requires repeated stimulation to attend or painful stimulation to make movements
  - ❏ 3 = Responds only with reflex motor or autonomic effects or totally unresponsive
- Ability to answer questions correctly
  - What is your age and what is the month?
  - Item 1b LOC—questions scoring
    - ❏ 0 = Answers both questions correctly
    - ❏ 1 = Answers one question correctly
    - ❏ 2 = Answers neither question correctly
  - Special scoring situations
    - ❏ Aphasic patients score a 2
    - ❏ Intubated patients or patients with language barrier or severe dysarthria score a 1

Fast Facts

Do not coach the patient. (Example: If it is December and the patient says November, do not ask what month Christmas is in.)

- Ability to follow commands
  - The patient is asked to open and close his or her eyes and grip and release both hands
  - Item 1c LOC—commands scoring
    - ❏ 0 = Performs both tasks correctly
    - ❏ 1 = Performs one task correctly
    - ❏ 2 = Performs neither task correctly
  - Special scoring situations
    - ❏ Rarely are these patients untestable
    - ❏ For patients who attempt to complete the commands but cannot because of weakness, credit is given
    - ❏ Patients with trauma, amputation, or other physical issues should be given one-step commands

Best Gaze

- Assessment
  - Awake patients

- ❏ Assess extraocular eye movements; only the horizontal movements are being assessed
- ❏ Assess by having the patient follow your finger or pen light
- ❏ Confused patients can be assessed using tracking
- ■ Unresponsive patients are assessed with oculocephalics
  - ❏ Normal response to oculocephalics is that eyes move in the *opposite* direction to head movement
  - ❏ Abnormal response to oculocephalics is that eyes are fixed and follow the direction the head is turned
- ■ Item 2: Best gaze scoring
  - ❏ 0 = Normal horizontal eye movements
  - ❏ 1 = Partial gaze palsy (abnormality in one or both eyes, but forced deviation is not present)
  - ❏ 2 = Forced deviation or total gaze paresis (not overcome with oculocephalic maneuver)

Fast Facts

Make sure to ask the patient or available historian about blindness or previous eye surgeries.

Visual Fields

- ■ Assessment
  - ■ The examiner stands approximately 2 feet away when possible; the patient is asked to look at the examiner's nose and trust his or her peripheral vision
    - ❏ Each eye is tested independently
    - ❏ The four quadrants are tested with each eye separately
  - ■ Can be tested using finger counting or blinks to threat/ movement to confrontation
- ■ Item 3: Visual fields scoring
  - ■ 0 = No visual loss
  - ■ 1 = Partial hemianopia, quadrantanopia
  - ■ 2 = Complete hemianopia
  - ■ 3 = Bilateral hemianopia = Blind

Facial Palsy

- ■ In this section it is okay to coach or pantomime
- ■ Awake patient

- Close eyes tightly: Observe for weakness of one eyelid
- Raise your eyebrows: Observe for forehead wrinkles
- Show me your teeth/smile with teeth: Observe for flattening of nasolabial fold or lower facial paralysis
- Unresponsive or confused patient
  - Observe facial grimace to noxious stimuli
  - Lightly touch nasal passages; observe facial movements
- Item 4: Facial palsy scoring
  - 0 = Normal symmetric movement
  - 1 = Minor paralysis (flattened nasolabial fold, asymmetric smile)
  - 2 = Partial paralysis (total or near total paralysis of lower face)
  - 3 = Complete paralysis of one or both sides of face (no movement in upper and lower face)
- Special situation scoring
  - Comatose patients, patients with bilateral paresis, or patients with unilateral upper and lower facial weakness receive a score of 3

Motor Arm

- Assessment: Hold both arms out and close your eyes
- Item 5: Motor arm scoring
  - 0 = No drift, able to hold arm in position for 10 seconds
  - 1 = Drifts down before 10 seconds but does not hit bed or other support
  - 2 = Some effort against gravity but cannot get to or maintain level; drifts down to bed but has some effort against gravity
  - 3 = Limb immediately falls, no effort against gravity; trace muscular contraction present in limb or can move arm on bed without raising
  - 4 = No movement
  - Untestable (UN) = Amputation, joint fusion
- Special situation scoring
  - Each limb is tested independently, starting with the nonparetic arm
  - You can help the patient get the limb in correct position, but he or she must be able to maintain the limb in that position without support
  - Count out loud—this will encourage continued effort

Motor Leg

- Assessment: Ask patient to lift and hold leg off bed ×5 seconds
- Item 6: Motor leg scoring
  - 0 = No drift, holds leg at 30 degrees position for full 5 seconds
  - 1 = Drifts down before 5 seconds, but leg does not hit bed or other support
  - 2 = Some effort against gravity, leg falls to bed before 5 seconds
  - 3 = Limb immediately falls, no effort against gravity; trace muscular contraction present in limb
  - 4 = No movement
  - UN = Amputation, joint fusion
- Special situation scoring
  - Make sure you assess for muscle contraction
  - You may assist the patient by lifting the leg, but then the patient must be able to maintain the position on his or her own, without support

Limb Ataxia

- Assessment: Ask the patient to touch your finger, and then touch his or her nose or perform heel to shin; each limb is tested independently
- Item 7: Limb ataxia scoring
  - 0 = Absent
  - 1 = Present in one limb
  - 2 = Present in two limbs
- Special situation scoring
  - If the patient cannot understand the exam or is paralyzed, the patient receives a score of 0
  - In a patient with mild ataxia, for which it is unclear whether the ataxia is only resultant from weakness, the patient receives a score of 0

Sensory

- Assessment: Sensory is assessed utilizing pinprick on the patient's face, arms, trunk, and legs. This is done in the same spot bilaterally to assess for equality and characterize differences if present. This should *not* be performed through clothing.
- Item 8: Sensory scoring
  - 0 = Normal, no sensory loss

- 1 = Mild to moderate sensory loss; aware of being touched but pinprick is less sharp on the affected side
- 2 = Severe to total sensory loss; no awareness of being touched
- Special situation scoring
  - Watch for grimacing or withdrawal from pinprick in obtunded or aphasic patients
  - Obtunded or aphasic patients typically score a 0 or 1
  - Comatose patients typically score a 2
  - Take note if preexisting sensory loss was present (as in a previous stroke) and only record new sensory loss

Fast Facts

Do not attempt to perform pinprick stimulation with blunt-tip needles or medication needles. If you do not have single-use "pins," a cotton swab or tongue depressor can be broken in half and safely substituted if a decent point is obtained.

Best Language

- Assessment: The language exam requires provided material in the NIHSS stroke booklet (see Appendix A), including the "cookie thief" picture, the naming card, and sentences
- Item 9: Best language scoring
  - 0 = No aphasia, normal fluency and comprehension
  - 1 = Mild to moderate aphasia, some obvious loss of fluency or comprehension with reduction of speech and/or compensation but able to communicate ideas
  - 2 = Severe aphasia, all communication is limited, examiner guesses at what is attempted to be communicated
  - 3 = Mute, global aphasia, no usable speech, no auditory comprehension; patient usually cannot follow any one-step commands
- Special situation scoring
  - To determine if a patient is a 1 or a 2, all material should be assessed; if the patient misses two thirds, the score is a 2
  - Visually impaired patients should use glasses if they have them; if their vision is still too impaired to see, you can place objects in their hands and ask them to identify them

■ Patients who cannot speak can be asked to point at objects on the naming card to assess comprehension

■ Intubated patients may be asked to write if alert enough

Fast Facts

"Hand"/"glove" or "feather"/"leaf" are often used interchangeably and should not be counted against the patient. It is not unusual for patients from outside the United States to be unable to identify a hammock. This also should not be counted against the patient.

Dysarthria

■ Assessment: Do *not* tell the patient you are assessing his or her speech; the patient should be asked to read words/phrases from the stroke book

■ Item 10: Dysarthria scoring
  ■ 0 = Normal
  ■ 1 = Mild to moderate, patient slurs some words or can be understood with some difficulty
  ■ 2 = Severe, patient's speech is so slurred that it cannot be understood, the patient is mute
  ■ UN = Intubated

■ Special situation scoring
  ■ Aphasic patients should be asked to repeat words after you say them
  ■ Comatose patients should score a 2

Extinction and Inattention

■ Assessment: Alternatively touch each side of the patient and ask the patient to identify which side you are touching; after this, touch both sides and ask which side you are touching

■ Item 11: Extinction and inattention scoring
  ■ 0 = No abnormality
  ■ 1 = Visual, tactile, auditory, spatial, or personal inattention or extinction to bilateral stimulation in one of the sensory modalities
  ■ 2 = Profound hemi-inattention or hemi-inattention to more than one modality

Table 2.2

NIHSS Items With Poor Interrater Reliability

Level of consciousness

Facial movement

Limb ataxia

Dysarthria

Neglect

NIHSS, National Institute of Health Stroke Scale.

- Special situation scoring
  - A patient who cannot recognize his or her own arm or only orients to one side should be scored a 2
  - Aphasic patients who attend to both sides receive a normal score
  - A patient with severe visual loss preventing visual double stimulation, but with normal cutaneous stimulation, receives a normal score
  - Neglect is scored only if present, so it is never untestable

LIMITATIONS OF THE NIHSS

The NIHSS is not useful in the identification or classification of posterior circulation strokes. These patients may have low NIHSS scores but still have a devastating outcome. Additionally, some NIHSS items have poor interrater reliability, which means that two examiners have potential to have high variation in scores (Table 2.2).

Bibliography

National Institute of Neurological Disorders and Stroke. (2006). *NIH stroke scale*. Retrieved from https://www.ninds.nih.gov/sites/default/files/NIH_Stroke_Scale_Booklet.pdf

3

Neurological Examination of the Comatose Patient

Neurological examination of the comatose patient can be particularly challenging because the patient cannot follow commands. Patients in a comatose state can have either a structural or a metabolic derangement. The goal of the exam of the comatose patient is to determine the likely cause of the coma.

In this chapter, you will learn how to:

- Define coma.
- Demonstrate examination strategies specific to the comatose patient.
- Discuss coma mimics and differentiate between true comatose state.

DEFINITION OF COMA

The term "coma" describes a pathologic state of unarousable unresponsiveness. The person is unable to be aroused and is unaware of his or her surroundings or condition. Comatose patients do not make any purposeful responses or movements. Arousal is dependent upon an intact ascending reticular activating system in the brainstem. Awareness typically resides in the cerebral cortices.

Fast Facts

Toxic metabolic encephalopathy is the most common cause of coma.

Some sources differentiate between light coma and deep coma. In light coma, the examiner can elicit a posturing motor response, whereas in deep coma the examiner is unable to elicit a response at all during examination of the motor system.

Fast Facts

A, B, Cs: Emergency treatment of the comatose patient includes prompt recognition and treatment of hypoxia, shock, herniation syndrome, and hypoglycemia, which all contribute to neuronal death.

EVALUATION OF COMA

The evaluation of coma includes many different components, including physical examination, neurological examination, laboratory findings, neuroimaging, and additional diagnostic studies. The etiology of coma may be clearer in some circumstances than others. This workup will help you identify the underlying cause of coma.

Physical Examination

A quick physical assessment of the patient should be performed immediately to ensure patient safety and determine whether the patient has an acute process that requires intervention. The examiner can very quickly observe vital signs, the general appearance of the patient, any spontaneous movements, and the respiratory pattern. This is also a good time to observe for track marks, toxidromes, and meningeal signs, all of which can help the examiner determine the cause of coma.

Easily fixable causes of coma should also be considered during the initial sweep. This includes blood glucose check to evaluate for

Table 3.1

Different Respiratory Patterns Commonly Seen in Coma; These Patterns May Help the Provider Localize the Area of Injury		
Name	**Pattern**	**Localization**
Sighing respirations and yawning	Often accompanied by drowsiness	Diffuse cerebral cortical dysfunction
Cheyne–Stokes respirations	Alternating cycle of hyperpnea and apnea	Diffuse bilateral cerebral involvement
Neurogenic hyperventilation	Sustained but regular, rapid, deep respirations	Midbrain and pons
Cluster breathing	Clusters of respirations irregular in frequency and amplitude with variable pauses between clusters	Pons
Ataxic breathing	Irregular in rate and volume	Medulla
Apneustic breathing	Prolonged pause at end of inspiration	Midpontine

hypoglycemia, which can be rapidly detected and treated. Thiamine should be given prior to glucose in patients at risk for nutritional deficiencies to prevent Wernicke's encephalopathy. Naloxone can be administered to patients when there is concern of opioid overdose.

Hypertension and bradycardia suggest the patient may have a herniation syndrome that requires immediate intervention. Respiratory patterns may help the examiner localize where the lesion is (Table 3.1). The examiner must also evaluate the patient's ability to protect his or her airway.

Neurological Examination

Many components of the neurological examination of the comatose patient are well covered in the general neurological examination (Chapter 1). For the purpose of this chapter, the examination will be limited specifically to comatose patients. The purpose of the neurological examination in comatose patients remains to identify causative factors or localize the lesion. Early on, it may be difficult to establish if the etiology of coma is metabolic or structural. When considering metabolic causes, a useful mnemonic is COATPEGS (carbon dioxide, oxygen, ammonia, temperature, pH, electrolytes, glucose, and serum osmolality).

The exam typically first establishes comatose state, followed by examination factors that help localize the lesion.

- Level of consciousness
- Glasgow Coma Scale (GCS)
  - GCS scores less than 8 are consistent with coma
  - GCS scores of 3 and 4 are generally associated with poor outcomes, including death or vegetative state
  - Limitations of the GCS
    - Patients who are locked-in receive low GCS scores and may be missed if relying only upon GCS scoring
    - Once a patient has a low GCS score, the score does not continue to reflect worsening status or subtle changes
    - Patients who are intubated receive a "T" or "1" for best verbal response, when the patient may be oriented, despite intubation
    - The GCS score is skewed toward motor response
- Full outline of unresponsiveness (FOUR) score
  - The FOUR score was developed to address some of the limitations of GCS. The FOUR score is also able to localize the area of injury more specifically than GCS.
  - The FOUR score measures four areas: eye response, motor response, brainstem reflexes, and respirations. For each area, the patient is scored 0, 1, 2, 3, or 4 (Table 3.2). The lowest score is 0 and is consistent with brain death. The highest score a patient can receive is 16.
  - The FOUR score
    - E: Eye response
      - Make at least three attempts to elicit the *best* possible response
      - In patients with significant periorbital edema or trauma, one eyelid can be opened in an attempt to elicit best response

Table 3.2

Scoring Criteria for the FOUR Score

Eye Response	Motor Response	Brainstem Reflexes	Respirations
4: Eyelids open or open/ track/blink to command	4: Thumbs-up, fist, or peace sign	4: Pupil and corneal reflexes are present	4: Nonintubated, regular breathing pattern
3: Eyelids open but do not track	3: Localizes to pain	3: One pupil fixed and dilated	3: Nonintubated, Cheyne–Stokes breathing pattern
2: Eyelids closed but open to loud noise or voice	2: Flexion response to pain	2: Pupil or corneal reflexes are absent	2: Nonintubated, irregular breathing pattern
1: Eyelids closed but open to pain	1: Extension response to pain	1: Pupil and corneal reflexes absent; cough present	1: Intubated, but initiates respirations over ventilator rate
0: Eyelids remain closed to pain	0: No response to pain or general- ized myoclonus status	0: Absent pupil, corneal, and cough reflex	0: Breathes at ventila- tor rate or apneic

FOUR, full outline of unresponsiveness.

- Determine if the patient can blink on command; if the patient can give two blinks on command, the patient may be locked-in
- M: Motor response
  - Score the best response
  - To achieve a score of 4, the patient must demonstrate a thumbs-up, fist, or peace sign; this can be accomplished with either hand
  - To achieve a 3, the patient must localize to the examiner's hand when noxious stimulus is applied
- B: Brainstem reflexes
  - Corneal reflexes should be examined by the instillation of two or three drops of sterile saline onto the cornea from a distance of 4 to 6 inches
  - Cotton swabs may also be used to assess corneal reflex; however, repeated examinations put the patient at risk for corneal trauma

- Cough reflex should only be assessed when both pupillary and corneal reflexes are absent
  - R: Respiration
    - The respiration score already takes into account whether the patient is intubated or not
    - In intubated patients, do not make any adjustments on the ventilator; simply observe the quality of patient-generated respirations
    - Ideally, the $PaCO_2$ is within normal limits during assessment
    - If the patient does not initiate spontaneous respirations, apnea testing may be required
- Mental status
  - Evaluate the patient's response to stimuli; comatose patients typically require noxious stimuli
    - Using your thumb, apply pressure to the bony superior roof of the orbital cavity
    - Press a pen or other solid substance strongly against the patient's nail bed
- Motor exam
  - Assess tone, reflexes, and posturing
    - Tone
    - Upper motor lesions often cause spasticity
  - Motor response may not be as helpful in localizing a structural brain lesion as other components of the exam
  - Patients with decorticate posturing are typically thought to have a better prognosis than patients with decerebrate posturing

Fast Facts

Note asymmetry in motor response. This is more likely to be associated with a structural cause of coma, rather than metabolic. This is not *always* the case though, as Todd's paralysis s/p seizure or even hypoglycemia can result in asymmetry of exam.

- Pupil exam (Table 3.3)
  - Assess shape, size, symmetry, and response to light
    - Metabolic coma: small pupils that react to light
      - In metabolic coma, the pupillary response to light is often the last brainstem reflex detected

Table 3.3

Pupil Responses and Localization of Pathology to Different Areas of the Brain

Location	Dark		Light		Description
Awake	●	●	⊙	⊙	Normal response
Metabolic; diencephalic	⊙	⊙	⊙	⊙	Small, reactive
Midbrain tectum	●	●	●	●	Unreactive, spontaneous hippus, midline
Midbrain tegmentum	◉	◉	◉	◉	Unreactive, irregular, midline, correctopia
Fascicular	●	●	●	⊙	Ipsilateral unresponsive and large
Pons	·	·	·	·	Pinpoint, responsive

▫ Unilateral hypothalamic damage: miosis (excessive constriction) and anhidrosis (decreased sweating) ipsilateral to the lesion
  • Commonly called Horner's syndrome

Fast Facts

Pupil light reflex dysfunction is rarely caused by metabolic abnormalities. Noteworthy exceptions include overdoses. If the eyes do not constrict to light reflex, 1% pilocarpine can be instilled in the affected eye. If the pupil is dilated as a result of anoxia, pilocarpine will cause miosis. If the dilation is pharmacologic iridoplegia, pilocarpine will have no effect.

■ Eye movements
  ▪ This cannot be assessed using voluntary eye movements, so oculocephalic and oculovestibular reflexes are tested.

- ❑ Oculocephalic: This is tested by holding the eyes open and rotating the head from side to side. The patient has an intact oculocephalic reflex if the eyes move in the opposite direction of the head. This is often called "doll's eyes." This indicates an intact brainstem. This reflex is often masked in the awake patient due to voluntary eye movements overcoming the reflexive eye movement. A pathologic response would be a forward fixed gaze.
- ❑ Ensure the patient has an intact C-spine prior to performing this maneuver.
- ❑ Oculovestibular: This reflex is often referred to as "cold calorics." This can be tested by infusing ice water into the ear canal. The recommended rate of instillation is 10 mL/min. It is common to see 50 mL of ice water instilled into the ear within seconds, though this is incorrect technique. The eyes should deviate toward the tested ear.
- ❑ Awake patient; COWS mnemonic: Cold—Opposite, Warm—Same
- ❑ Comatose patient is opposite: Warm—Opposite, Cold—Same
- ❑ Ensure the patient has an intact ear canal prior to performing this maneuver
- ❑ Allow 5 minutes between testing ears so that the oculovestibular system can equilibrate

Fast Facts

The presence of nystagmus during cold calorics testing suggests that the patient is conscious.

- Corneal reflex
  - Loss is a late sign in coma
  - Corneal reflex: Unilateral loss may indicate structural lesion to facial or trigeminal nerve
  - Bell's phenomenon: Eyes roll upward in a patient with an intact upper pons and midbrain
  - Contact lens wearers typically have diminished corneal reflexes
- Gag reflex
  - May be absent in normal people

History

History is an important part of the evaluation of coma. The time of deterioration can provide valuable clues as to what may be the etiology of coma. An abrupt decline is more likely to be caused by stroke, seizure, or cardiac event. A gradual decline occurs more often with metabolic or infectious processes. Other information to gather includes medications, exposures, and drug and alcohol history.

INVESTIGATIONS

After your neurological examination establishes coma and you obtain a thorough history, you may start to have a hypothesis regarding whether the coma is metabolic or structural. Oftentimes, this remains unestablished and additional information is needed.

- Suggested laboratory tests
  - Bedside glucose
  - Complete blood count (CBC)
  - Chemistry
  - Toxicology screening
    - Ethanol (ETOH)
    - Urine toxicology screen
- Suggested neuroimaging
  - CT imaging
    - Noncontrast head CT
      - Can quickly identify stroke, tumor, hydrocephalus
    - CT angiography (CTA) and CT perfusion (CTP)
      - Obtain if concerned about ischemic stroke
      - Particularly useful for basilar artery occlusion
    - CT with and without contrast
      - Useful if concern about central nervous system (CNS) infection, such as abscess or extra-axial fluid collection
  - MRI
    - Is sometimes used urgently in place of CTA/CTP when suspicion for hyperacute ischemic stroke exists
    - Otherwise, used nonacutely and can provide additional information when no other clear source of coma is identified
- Other diagnostics
  - Lumbar puncture (LP)
    - Indications/suspicions
      - CNS infection
      - Autoimmune/neuroinflammatory disorders
      - CNS involvement of malignancies
      - Concern for subarachnoid hemorrhage (SAH) in setting of normal CT scan

- EEG
  - Indications
    - Observed seizure without return to baseline
    - History of epilepsy, seizures
    - Subtle unexplained movements
  - Often will obtain 20-minute EEG first and then make determination whether to continue

COMA MIMICS

- Hysterical coma; catatonic state
  - Can be quite convincing, including no response to noxious stimuli
  - Tests to differentiate from true coma
    - EEG: will be normal and show an alert state
    - Oculovestibular testing: presence of nystagmus
- Locked-in syndrome
  - The patient has lost all ability to move but does not have impairment of consciousness
    - Can occur with myasthenia gravis, Guillain–Barré syndrome, or certain drugs/medications
      - History is usually obvious
    - Can occur with damage to the base of the pons
      - Can occur as a result of hemorrhage, infarction, or acute myelin destruction, such as central pontine myelinolysis (CPM)
      - Usually is not obvious and is easily missed unless the examiner asks the patient to look up and down
      - The patient becomes acutely unresponsive and is unable to move except vertical eye movements and eye opening systems

Bibliography

Cadena, R., & Sarwal, A. (2017). Emergency neurological life support: Approach to the patient with coma. *Neurocritical Care, 17*(Suppl. 1), S69–S75. doi:10.1007/s12028-017-0452-1

Wijdicks, E. F. (2016). *The practice of emergency and critical care neurology* (2nd ed.). New York, NY: Oxford University Press. doi:10.1093/med/9780190259556.001.0001

Wijdicks, E. F., Bamlet, W. R., Maramattom, B. V., Manno, E. M., & McClelland, R. L. (2005). Validation of a new coma scale: The FOUR score. *Annals of Neurology, 58*(4), 585–593. doi:10.1002/ana.20611

4

Intracranial Hypertension

It is essential to understand the concept of intracranial hypertension to realize the consequences of many of the other disorders detailed within this book. Intracranial pressure (ICP) can rise transiently without becoming pathologic (e.g., a sneeze). In sustained increased ICP, brain herniation can occur, which can lead to severe morbidity and death. This chapter will explain the concept of ICP, herniation, and the ways to manage acute rise in ICP.

In this chapter, you will learn how to:

- Explain the Monro–Kellie doctrine and its application to ICP.
- Describe brain herniation syndromes.
- Detail measurement and treatment strategies to decrease ICP.

PATHOPHYSIOLOGY

The Monro–Kellie doctrine describes the skull as being a fixed box containing brain tissue, cerebrospinal fluid (CSF), and blood. If there is an increase in any one of these components, there must be a compensatory change in another in order to prevent an increase in pressure. These components are very limited in the amount that they can compensate; therefore, any space-occupying lesion (hemorrhage, tumor), edema, or increase in CSF can result in increased pressure, which may subsequently shift structures into an opening or into an adjacent space that they do not typically occupy (herniation).

INTRACRANIAL HYPERTENSION

- Normal ICP
  - 5 to 15 mmHg, but anything less than 20mmHg is nonpathologic.
- ICP greater than 20 mmHg
  - Reduces cerebral perfusion pressure (CPP)
  - Can cause ischemic brain injury
- CPP
  - CPP is the difference between mean arterial pressure (MAP) and ICP
  - Autoregulation refers to the brain's ability to maintain constant cerebral blood flow (CBF) over a range of CPP (60–150 mmHg)
    - May be impaired or absent in the injured brain
  - CPP less than 60 mmHg decreases CBF and can lead to ischemic brain injury
  - CPP greater than 150 mmHg can lead to cerebral edema
  - CPP may be more important than ICP measurement in outcomes

Causes

- Space-occupying lesion
  - Intracranial blood
    - Epidural
    - Subdural
    - Subarachnoid
    - Intraparenchymal
  - Brain tumor
  - Brain abscess
- Cerebral edema (Table 4.1)
  - Cytotoxic
    - Intracellular edema
    - Intact blood–brain barrier
  - Vasogenic
    - Extracellular edema
    - Loss of intact blood–brain barrier
    - Associated with brain tumor or inflammation disorder
- CSF accumulation

Table 4.1

Differentiation of Cytotoxic From Vasogenic Edema

Differences in Cerebral Edema

Cytotoxic	Vasogenic
Intracellular	Extracellular
Blood–brain barrier intact	Blood–brain barrier nonintact
Restrict diffusion pattern on MRI	MRI does not have restricted diffusion pattern
Loss of gray–white differentiation	Accentuation of gray–white differentiation
Predominantly affects gray matter	Predominantly affects white matter
Following stroke or hypoxic encephalopathy	Brain tumors
Osmotherapy (mannitol, 23.4% NS)	Steroids (Decadron)

NS, normal saline.

Fast Facts

Approximately 20 mL of CSF is produced every hour.

- Hydrocephalus
  - Accumulation of CSF causing widening of the ventricles
  - Types of hydrocephalus
    - Communicating
      - CSF is blocked after exiting ventricles but can still flow between ventricles
      - Causes
        - Congenital
    - Noncommunicating/obstructive
      - CSF is blocked along the path connecting the ventricles
      - Causes
        - Subarachnoid hemorrhage
        - Aqueductal stenosis
    - Hydrocephalus ex vacuo
      - Compensatory enlargement of the ventricles
      - Brain tissue shrinks following stroke or traumatic brain injury
    - Normal pressure hydrocephalus
      - Hydrocephalus not associated with increased ICP

- Hygroma
  - CSF collection without blood
  - Most commonly subdural
  - Often seen in elderly after trauma or subdural hematoma or in children after infection
- Pneumocephalus
  - Air trapped in the intracranial vault
  - Can cause displacement and compression of brain tissue
  - Causes
    - Following neurosurgery
    - Following ear, nose, and throat (ENT) surgery
    - Rarely: spontaneously
  - Symptoms
    - Headache
    - Symptoms of increased ICP
    - Altered level of consciousness
    - Focal findings based upon mass effect
  - CT findings (Figure 4.1)
    - Anechoic area with adjacent compression or flattening of sulci
    - Mount Fuji sign in tension pneumocephalus
  - Treatment
    - Conservative: allow to reabsorb over time

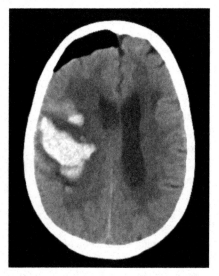

Figure 4.1 Pneumocephalus. (The dark area in the left upper portion of the intracranial vault depicts pneumocephalus.)

- Oxygen therapy to wash out nitrogen
  - Most protocols provide 100% supplemental oxygen
    - Alternating or continuous
    - 8 to 24 hours
    - Ventilator, nonrebreather, or high-flow nasal cannula
  - Surgical decompression in extreme cases
- Valsalva maneuver
  - Coughing
  - Sneezing

BRAIN HERNIATION

- Supratentorial
  - Uncal transtentorial herniation
    - Uncinate process of the temporal lobe herniates into the anterior opening of the tentorium cerebelli
    - Compresses the posterior cerebral artery as it crosses the tentorium and causes posterior cerebral artery (PCA) territory infarct
  - Central tentorial herniation
    - Thalamic region herniates downward through the opening of the tentorium cerebelli
  - Subfalcine herniation
    - Cingulate gyrus displaces across the midline and beneath the falx
  - Transcalvarial herniation
    - External herniation
    - Brain displaces through skull defect (fracture or postcraniectomy)
- Infratentorial
  - Upward transtentorial herniation
    - Reverse coning
    - Posterior fossa mass displaces upward
    - Most commonly occurs when external ventricular drain (EVD) is placed supratentorial for ICP monitoring or hydrocephalus and posterior fossa contents are pulled upward
  - Tonsillar or foraminal herniation
    - Cerebellar tonsils displace downward through the foramen magnum

Signs and Symptoms

- Physical exam findings
  - Headache
    - Continuous
    - May be worse in the morning (after lying flat all night)
  - Emesis
    - Often not preceded by nausea
    - Projectile
  - Altered mental status
    - Confusion
    - Loss of consciousness
    - Coma
  - Seizures
  - Vision changes
  - Pupil changes
- Vital signs abnormalities
  - Cushing's triad: widened pulse pressure, bradycardia, irregular respirations
  - Hypertension
  - Bradycardia
  - Respiratory pattern changes
  - Shallow breathing
- CT features of increased ICP
  - Effacement of basal cisterns
  - Loss of sulci
  - Loss of gray–white differentiation
  - Midline shift
  - Herniation syndromes

DIAGNOSIS OF INCREASED ICP

- ICP monitors
  - EVD
    - EVD is the gold standard ICP monitor because it is the only device that can both monitor and treat elevations of ICP
    - Typically leveled at tragus
      - Many institutions will also level arterial lines at the tragus to calculate CPP when an EVD is in place
    - ICP waveform can indicate cerebral compliance (Figure 4.2)
      - P1—percussion wave—arterial pulsation

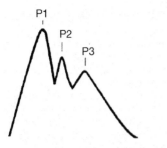
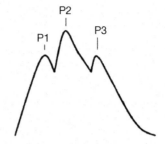

Normal ICP waveform   Abnormal noncompliant ICP waveform

Figure 4.2 Demonstration of a normal ICP waveform and an ICP waveform with P2 prominence, suggestive of poor intracranial compliance.
ICP, intracranial pressure.
Illustration: Nicholas McLaughlin.

- P2—tidal wave—cerebral compliance
- P3—dicrotic wave—venous pulsation
- Normal ICP is less than 20 mmHg
  - ICP may increase during times of high pressure, such as sneezing or coughing, but is not a concern unless it does not return to less than 20 mmHg
  - ICP sustaining greater than 20 mmHg for 5 or more minutes should be addressed

Fast Facts

A normal ICP waveform follows a step-like progression, in which the amplitude of P1 is greater than P2, which is greater than P3 (Figure 4.2).

- Fiberoptic catheter
  - Sensor located within the catheter tip
  - May be placed intraparenchymally or in the ventricle
- Bolt
  - Typically placed between the arachnoid membrane and cerebral cortex
- Transcranial Doppler
  - Measures CBF
  - Can evaluate cerebral compliance
  - Noninvasive
  - Posterior circulation can be obtained; however it is more difficult and not commonly done

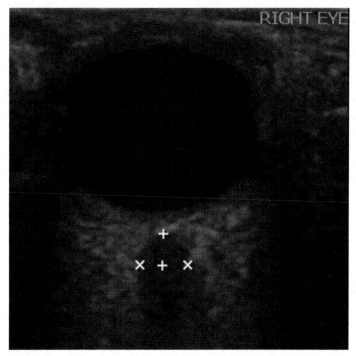

Figure 4.3 Demonstration of ultrasound insonation of the optic nerve sheath with measurement across the diameter.

- Optic nerve sheath diameter (Figure 4.3)
  - Ultrasound
    - Dilation of the optic nerve sheath beyond 0.5 cm has been associated with an ICP greater than 20 mmHg
    - Quick, noninvasive
    - Unlikely to correlate with changes in pressure in the infratentorium

NURSING INTERVENTIONS

- Positioning: Assure optimal venous return from the brain
  - Head of bed at 30 degrees
  - Midline neutral positioning
  - Avoid any venous compression
- Observe for signs of sleep apnea
  - If CO_2 increases during apneic periods, it is often accompanied by increased ICP

MEDICAL INTERVENTIONS

- Optimize oxygen delivery
  - PaO_2
  - Treat anemia
- Maintain CPP greater than 60 mmHg
  - Fluids
  - Vasopressors

Fast Facts

Do not administer dextrose solutions. They decrease plasma osmolality and increase water content within brain tissue.

- Cerebral vasoconstriction avoidance
  - Goal $PaCO_2$ of 35 to 45 mmHg

Fast Facts

CO_2 dilates cerebral vasculature, which increases intracranial blood volume and increases ICP. Acutely, hyperventilation can be used to help bring down ICP; however long-term use of hyperventilation should be avoided, as the vasoconstriction that occurs could reduce CBF to the point of ischemia.

- Decrease cerebral metabolic rate
  - Pain control
  - Sedation
  - Neuromuscular blockade
  - Treat seizures
  - Hyperthermia avoidance
- Medication—osmotherapy
  - Mannitol (0.25–1 g/kg)
    - Target: serum osmolality of 300 to 320 mOsm/kg
    - Stop administration for any serum osmolality greater than 330 mOsm/kg
    - Can be given peripherally
    - Standard dose is 100 g of 20% mannitol

- Hypertonic saline (23.4%)
  - Often given in volumes of 15 to 30 mL at a time
  - Target: serum Na of 145 to 155 mEq
  - Must be given via a central line
  - Also called "hot salts"
- Hypertonic saline (3%)
  - Can be given carefully through a peripheral line at a low rate
    - Monitor for phlebitis
    - Cannot run with any other medications
    - Do not exceed rate of 30 mL/hr
    - If extending infusions or giving at an increased rate, place central venous access
  - Used to slowly drive sodium to goal range
- Consider repeat imaging
  - Worsening edema
  - Increasing hematoma, lesion size
  - Accumulating hydrocephalus

NEUROSURGICAL INTERVENTIONS

- Reduction of intracranial volume
  - EVD placement
  - Hematoma evacuation
  - Tumor debulking
- Opening the cranial vault to allow expansion
  - Decompressive craniectomy
    - Controversial, as it may not reduce morbidity or avoid death

Bibliography

Wijdicks, E. F. (2016). *The practice of emergency and critical care neurology* (2nd ed.). New York, NY: Oxford University Press. doi:10.1093/med/9780190259556.001.0001

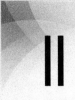

Stroke

5

Ischemic Stroke

Ischemic stroke is a leading cause of disability and death in the United States. It is caused by a disruption of blood flow to the brain due to thrombus or embolus. Not all patients admitted to the hospital with ischemic stroke require critical care; however, all patients who present as a possible ischemic stroke (commonly called "stroke alert" or "code stroke") require immediate assessment for diagnosis and intervention to decrease disability and death.

In this chapter, you will learn how to:

- Describe stroke risk factors.
- Discuss the etiology and pathophysiology of ischemic stroke.
- Describe typical exam findings associated with common stroke symptoms.

PATHOPHYSIOLOGY OF STROKE

- Cerebral circulation
  - Anterior circulation is supplied by the internal carotid arteries
  - Posterior circulation is supplied by the vertebral arteries
  - Intracranial cerebral circulation takes place via the circle of Willis (Figure 5.1)
- Risk factors
  - Modifiable
    - Lifestyle factors

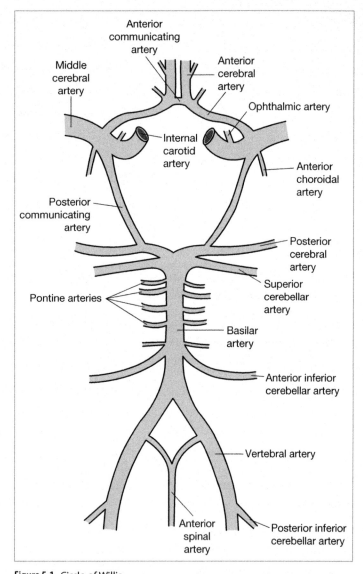

Figure 5.1 Circle of Willis.

Source: Morrison, K. (2018). *Fast facts for stroke care nursing: An expert care guide* (2nd ed., p. 20). New York, NY: Springer Publishing.

Table 5.1

Some Common Nonmodifiable and Modifiable Risk Factors for Stroke	
Nonmodifiable	**Modifiable**
Age—two-thirds ischemic CVA over age of 65	Hypertension
Women > men	Alcohol use
African Americans	Cocaine use
Family history of stroke	High-fat diet
Genetics—lipid metabolism, thrombosis, etc.	Smoking

CVA, cerebrovascular accident.

- Nonmodifiable
- Heart disease is an important risk factor for stroke and itself has components of both modifiable and nonmodifiable risk factors (Table 5.1)

Fast Facts

Atrial fibrillation is responsible for about 20% of all strokes; incidence increases with age.

TYPES OF ISCHEMIC STROKE

Transient Ischemic Attack

- Definition
  - Transient ischemic attack (TIA): a reduction of cerebral blood flow to one focal region that does not cause tissue death

Fast Facts

Never assume that stroke symptoms are a TIA—all stroke symptoms should be treated as a stroke unless proven otherwise. All TIAs should be treated as a medical emergency.

- Pathophysiology
  - TIAs are likely due to microemboli that temporarily block the blood flow

- Signs and symptoms
  - Due to the location of the blockage and the brain experiencing ischemia
  - Symptoms typically last less than 1 hour but can persist significantly longer
- Prognosis
  - One third of individuals who have a TIA will progress to an ischemic stroke; one third will experience additional TIAs and one third will never experience another event

Table 5.2

ABCD² Score			
	0	1	2
Age ≥ 60 years	No	Yes	
BP ≥ 140/90 mmHg (Initial BP)	No	Yes	
Clinical features of TIA	Other symptoms	Speech disturbance without weakness	Unilateral weakness
Duration of symptoms	<10 minutes	10–59 minutes	≥60 minutes
History of diabetes	No	Yes	

Fast Facts

The ABCD² score helps estimate subsequent stroke probability and can help providers determine whether stroke workup should be done in an inpatient or outpatient setting. An ABCD² score of 2 or less is associated with a less than 1% chance of stroke in the next week (Table 5.2).

Thrombotic Stroke

- Definition
  - Blockage of cerebral blood flow resultant from thrombosis or narrowing of the blood vessel that *does* cause tissue death/ infarction
  - Thrombotic stroke is the most common cause of stroke (~60%)
- Pathophysiology
  - The major cause of ischemic stroke is atherosclerosis, which leads to thrombus formation

- Can result in occlusion leading to infarction
- Can contribute to emboli
- Injury to a vessel wall can lead to the formation of blood clots/occlusion

Fast Facts

Hypertension and diabetes mellitus are both risk factors for thrombotic stroke due to their role in the development of atherosclerotic plaque.

- Signs and symptoms
  - Again, signs and symptoms are based upon the location of thrombosis and area of the brain that particular vessel feeds
  - Other factors that influence signs and symptoms and prognosis include
    - Onset time
    - Size of affected area
    - Presence of collateral circulation

Fast Facts

Collateral circulation is very important in ischemic stroke. If the main blood supply for a certain area of the brain is blocked, collateral vessels may be able to provide enough circulation to prevent complete infarction.

- Typically not associated with decreased level of consciousness
  - Exceptions to this include
    - Brainstem stroke
    - Seizures
    - Significant mass effect with increased intracranial pressure (ICP)
    - Hemorrhage
- Symptoms may progress over the first 72 hours as a result of increasing cerebral edema and infarction
- Prognosis
  - Variable
  - Dependent upon the amount of brain tissue deprived of blood supply

Embolic Stroke

- Definition
  - Blockage of cerebral blood flow resultant from embolus occluding a cerebral artery blood vessel that *does* cause tissue death/infarction
  - Embolic stroke is the second-most common cause of stroke (~24%)
- Pathophysiology
  - A major cause of embolic stroke in older adult is still atherosclerosis
    - Atherosclerotic plaque breaks off and eventually lodges in a cerebral artery
    - Rheumatic heart disease is a common cause in young or middle-aged adults
  - Can affect any age group
  - Sudden onset and may or may not be related to activity
  - Because of the fast onset, collateral circulation typically does not develop
- Signs and symptoms
  - Sudden onset
  - May or may not be related to activity
  - Headache is common
  - Neurological deficits are severe and rapidly progressive
    - May be temporary if embolus breaks up and allows blood to flow, but smaller emboli continue to travel until they become lodged in smaller distal vessels
  - Typically remain conscious
- Prognosis
  - Recurrence is common
  - Underlying cause needs aggressive treatment

CLINICAL MANIFESTATIONS OF STROKE

- Artery occluded and location of occlusion dictate dysfunction (Table 5.3)
  - Results from neural tissue destruction as result of hypoperfusion
  - Time of onset and duration of ischemia
- National Institute of Health Stroke Scale (NIHSS)
  - Quantitative assessment scale
    - Grades severity of stroke
    - Associated with patient outcomes
  - *See previous chapters for more details*

Table 5.3

Deficits That May Be Seen Dependent Upon the Vascular Region Affected by Stroke

ACA	MCA	PCA	Vertebrobasilar	Lacunar
Frontal lobe function	Upper extremity motor strip	Vision and thought	Difficult to localize; vague	Pure motor or sensory
Contralateral weakness (leg > arm)	Contralateral hemiparesis (arm > leg)	Altered mental status	Syncope, vertigo	Ataxic, hemiparetic strokes
Speech perseveration	Receptive or expressive aphasia(if lesion on dominant hemisphere)	Memory impairment	Ipsilateral cranial nerve deficits	No impairment of level of consciousness, speech, memory, or cognition
Grasp, rooting reflexes/primitive reflexes	Gaze preference toward lesion	Cortical blindness	Contralateral motor deficits	—
Disinhibition; impaired judgment	Agnosia	Visual agnosia	Nystagmus, double vision	—
Contralateral cortical sensory deficits	Ipsilateral hemianopia	Contralateral homonymous hemianopia	Dysphagia, dysarthria	—
Gait apraxia	Contralateral hypesthesia	—	Facial hypesthesia	—
Urinary incontinence	Neglect, inattention, extinction of double stimulation (with non-dominant hemisphere lesions)	—	Visual field deficits Ataxia	—

ACA, anterior cerebral artery; MCA, middle cerebral artery; PCA, posterior cerebral artery.

- Level of consciousness
- Cranial nerves
  - *See previous chapters*
- Motor function
  - Frequent motor deficits include
    - Akinesia—loss of purposeful movement
    - Decreased muscle tone
    - Hyporeflexia and then hyperreflexia
    - Initial flaccidity
      - Related to nerve damage
      - May last days to weeks
    - Spasticity following flaccid stage
      - Related to upper motor neuron interruptions

Fast Facts

Because the pyramidal pathway crosses at the level of the medulla, a lesion on one side of the brain affects motor function on the opposite side of the body (contralateral).

- Sensory function
- Cerebellar function
- Language
  - Aphasia
    - Occurs with the stroke affecting language centers in the dominant hemisphere
      - Receptive—loss of language comprehension
      - Expressive—loss of language production
      - Global—both receptive and expressive; typically unable to communicate
  - Dysphasia
    - Impaired language
    - Different from dysarthria, as there is not a *complete* loss
    - Often occurs with dysarthria
      - Nonfluent
        - Minimal speech activity
        - Slow speech
      - Fluent
        - Speech present
        - Contains little meaningful communication

- Receptive
  - ○ Comprehension affected
    - – Localizes to Wernicke's area
      - ◇ Left temporal lobe
- Expressive
  - ○ Cannot express thoughts
    - – Localizes to Broca's area
      - ◇ Left frontal lobe
- Dysarthria
  - ❏ Muscular control of speech/swallowing
  - ❏ Swallow must be evaluated prior to oral intake

DIAGNOSTIC STUDIES

- Neuroimaging
  - Noncontrast CT scan
    - ❏ Complete as soon as possible
    - ❏ Goal less than 25 minutes from presentation
    - ❏ Rule out mimics, such as lesion or intracerebral hemorrhage
    - ❏ Subjective measurement of infarct/edema
    - ❏ Middle cerebral artery (MCA) sign may be present
      - Appears as hyperdensity along MCA
      - Earliest visible sign of MCA infarction, but not always present
      - Alberta Stroke Program Early CT Score (ASPECTS) can be calculated from CT and is useful in identifying patients with high likelihood of poor functional outcome
        - ○ Requires certain level of expertise
        - ○ Relies upon identification of ischemia

Fast Facts

If greater than one third of the vascular territory is infarcted, then the patient typically is not considered a good candidate for intervention.

- MRI
  - ❏ Can be used for initial screening
  - ❏ Increased sensitivity and specificity in diagnosis of acute ischemic stroke as compared to noncontrast CT
  - ❏ Higher resolution with clearer images
    - Particularly diffusion MRI

❑ Many contraindications and limitations
  • Time-consuming
  • Less available
  • More expensive
  • Cannot be used in patients with metallic implants or foreign bodies
  • Weight restrictions
▪ Cerebral CT angiography (CTA) and CT perfusion (CTP)
  ❑ CTA: identifies occlusion
  ❑ CTP: evaluates size of infarction and area of penumbra
    • Mismatch: refers to cerebral blood flow (CBF) or mass transit time (MTT) abnormalities, whose area is greater than the core of the infarcted area (Tables 5.4 & 5.5).
      ○ Mismatch indicates penumbra (Figure 5.3), which refers to potentially reversible ischemia, as opposed to infarcted tissue

Table 5.4

Definitions

Important Measurements on CTP

	Definition	Units of Measurement	
CBF	Rate of blood flow through cerebral vasculature	mL/100 g/min	Decreased CBF identifies penumbra
CBV	Volume of blood flow	mL/100 g	Identifies core of infarcted tissue
MTT	Time required for blood to pass through the tissue	seconds	Increased MTT identifies penumbra

CBF, cerebral blood flow; CBV, cerebral blood volume; CTP, computed tomography perfusion; MTT, mean transit time.

Table 5.5

CBF Values' Definition Reference

	Range (mL/100 g/min)
Normal	55–110
Oligemia	23–44
Ischemia	10–22
Infarction	<10

CBF, cerebral blood flow.

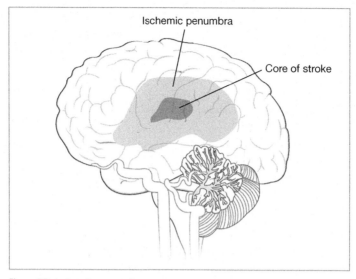

Figure 5.2 Ischemic penumbra.
Source: Morrison, K. (2018) *Fast facts for stroke care nursing: An expert care guide* (2nd ed., p. 33). New York, NY: Springer Publishing.

Fast Facts

CTP requires an 18-gauge intravenous (IV) catheter in the antecubital vein to deliver contrast agent at the appropriate speed. Many triple lumen catheters will *not* work for this purpose.

MANAGEMENT

- Medication
  - Tissue plasminogen activator (tPA)
    - Hallmark of medical management
    - Only Food and Drug Administration (FDA) approved therapy for treatment of acute ischemic stroke
    - Recommended to administer in patients who meet National Institute of Neurological Disorders and Stroke (NINDS) inclusion/exclusion criteria within 3 hours (Table 5.6)

Table 5.6

IV tPA Inclusion/Exclusion Criteria

Inclusion Criteria

Diagnosis of ischemic stroke

Onset within 4.5 hr before initiation of tPA (onset can be defined as last-known normal if exact time unknown)

18 years old or older

Exclusion Criteria

Clinical: symptoms suggestive of subarachnoid hemorrhage, persistent hypertension (SBP ≥185 mmHg or DBP ≥110 mmHg), serum glucose <50 mg/dL, active internal bleeding, acute bleeding diatheses

Hematologic: platelet count 1.7 or PT >15 sec, heparin use within 48 hr with an abnormally elevated aPTT, current use of a direct thrombin inhibitor or direct factor Xa inhibitor with evidence of prolonged bleeding times

Historical: stroke or head trauma within 3 months, previous intracranial hemorrhage, intracranial neoplasm, arteriovenous malformation or aneurysm, recent intracranial or spinal surgery, arterial puncture at a noncompressible site within 7 days

Head CT scan: evidence of hemorrhage, extensive regions of obvious hypodensity consistent with irreversible infarction

Relative Exclusions

Minor or isolated neurological signs

Rapid improving symptoms

Major surgery or trauma within 14 days

Gastrointestinal or urinary tract bleeding within 21 days

Myocardial infarction within 3 months

Seizure at stroke onset with postictal state

Pregnancy

Additional Relative Exclusions for 3–4.5 hr From Onset Treatment Window

Age >80 years

Oral anticoagulant use

Severe stroke as defined as NIHSS score >25

Combination of previous ischemic stroke and diabetes mellitus

aPTT, activated partial thromboplastin time; DBP, diastolic blood pressure; INR, international normalized ratio; NIHSS, National Institutes of Health Stroke Scale; SBP, systolic blood pressure; tPA, tissue plasminogen activator.

Fast Facts

If the patient has any of the following persistent neurological deficits—complete hemianopia, severe aphasia, visual or sensory extinction, weakness preventing antigravity movement, or National Institutes of Health Stroke Scale (NIHSS) score greater than 5—administration of tPA should be considered despite relative contraindications.

- How to administer IV tPA
  - Patient must have two peripheral IV catheters
  - Patient must have accurate weight
  - Dose: 0.9 mg/kg for a maximum dose of 90 mg
    - Ten percent is given as a bolus over 1 minute
    - Rest of the dose is given over 1 hour
    - *Stop if there is any neurological deterioration*
  - Complications include bleeding and angioedema
    - tPA can be reversed with cryoprecipitate or antifibrinolytics
    - Angioedema can be managed with high-dose steroids, diphenhydramine, and intubation, if indicated

Fast Facts

If a patient is going to receive tPA, consider the need for additional lines/tubes, such as Foley catheter or nasogastric tube (NGT), prior to administration. Please note that the need for these lines should *not* in any way delay the administration of tPA.

- Blood pressure control
  - Hypertension is common and needs to be well controlled in the acute phase
  - Blood pressure parameters vary based upon whether the patient has received tPA or endovascular therapy
    - If patient will receive tPA
      - Blood pressure (BP) must be less than 185/110 mmHg to be a candidate

- If patient *has* received tPA
  - BP goal less than 180/105 mmHg
  - Note: This is different than the pre-tPA goal
- If patient does *not* receive tPA or endovascular therapy
  - BP goal less than 220/120 mmHg
- Medications
  - Labetalol 10 to 20 mg IV q15m
  - Hydralazine 10 to 20 mg IV q4h
    - Watch for reflex tachycardia
  - Calcium channel blocker infusions
    - Nicardipine
      - Dose 5 to 15 mg/hr
      - High intravascular volume
    - Clevidipine
      - Dose variable, 1 to 21 mg/hr
      - Lipid based
- Antiplatelet drug therapy
  - Should be given to most patients with acute ischemic stroke or TIA
    - Aspirin
      - 160 to 325 mg/day
      - Reduced risk of early recurrent ischemic stroke
- Dual antiplatelet therapy
  - Given to patients with symptomatic large intracranial artery atherosclerotic stenosis, though risk of bleeding versus benefit of stroke prevention should be considered prior to prescription
    - Aspirin and Plavix for 90 days
    - Followed by monotherapy with aspirin

Fast Facts

If a patient does receive tPA, he or she should not receive anticoagulation or antiplatelet therapy until 24 hours have passed.

- Secondary stroke prevention
  - Statin therapy
    - Reduces risk of recurrent ischemic stroke
  - Selective serotonin-reuptake inhibitors (SSRIs)
    - May improve motor recovery and reduce dependency regardless of depression

- Neurosurgical intervention
  - Endovascular thrombectomy
    - Consider for patients who do not improve by 4 or more points on NIHSS score after IV tPA or do not meet IV tPA inclusion criteria and have a large-vessel occlusion
      - Intra-arterial tPA can be administered up to 6 hours after last known normal
      - Mechanical thrombectomy can be attempted up to 8 hours after last known normal
- Supportive care
  - Initial priority to airway, breathing, and circulation
  - Ensure euvolemic state
    - If requires hydration, recommend isotonic solution, such as normal saline or lactated Ringer's
  - Glucose control
    - Goal 140 to 180 mmHg
    - Avoid hypoglycemia
  - Normothermia
    - Aggressive avoidance of hyperthermia

COMPLICATIONS OF ISCHEMIC STROKE

- Cerebral edema
  - Malignant hemispheric stroke
    - Large stroke ~two-thirds of MCA or combined anterior cerebral artery (ACA)/MCA territory, or greater than 100 mL volume
      - Require more supportive care
      - Increased risk of hemorrhagic conversion
      - Mortality benefit when decompressive hemicraniectomy occurs within 48 hours; however, worse functional outcomes
  - See Chapter 4 for specific guidelines regarding cerebral edema and increased ICP management.
- Hemorrhagic conversion
  - For patient deterioration during or after tPA administration
    - *Immediately stop infusion*
    - Obtain stat CT
    - Obtain stat labs prothrombin time (PT)/international normalized ratio (INR), partial thromboplastin time (PTT), platelets, fibrinogen, type and cross
    - Consider administration of cryoprecipitate

Patients with higher NIHSS scores are more likely to develop symptomatic hemorrhagic conversion after receiving tPA.

Bibliography

Jauch, E. C., Saver, J. L., Adams, H. P. Jr., Bruno, A., Connors, J. J., Demaerschalk, B. M., . . . Yonas, H. (2013). Guidelines for the early management of patients with acute ischemic stroke: A guideline for healthcare professionals from the American Heart Association/American Stroke Association. *Stroke, 44*, 870–947. doi:10.1161/STR.0b013e318284056a

Morrison, K. (2018). *Fast facts for stroke care nursing: An expert care guide in a nutshell* (2nd ed.). New York, NY: Springer Publishing.

Powers, W. J., Derdeyn, C. P., Biller, J., Coffey, C. S., Hoh, B. L., Jauch, E. C., . . . Yavagal, D. R. (2015). American Heart Association/American Stroke Association focused update of the 2013 guidelines for the early management of patients with acute ischemic stroke regarding endovascular treatment. *Stroke, 46*, 3020–3035. doi:10.1161/STR.0000000000000074

Summers, D., Leonard, A., Wentworth, D., Saver, J. L., Simpson, J., Spilker, J. A., Hock, N., . . . Mitchell, P. H. (2009). Comprehensive overview of nursing and interdisciplinary care of the acute ischemic stroke patient: A scientific statement from the American Heart Association. *Stroke, 40*(8), 2911–2944. doi:10.1161/STROKEAHA.109.192362

6

Hemorrhagic Stroke

Hemorrhagic stroke is the second-most common cause of stroke; however, it is associated with higher mortality. Commonly known as intracranial hemorrhage (ICH), this occurs when there is spontaneous bleeding into the brain parenchyma, not resultant from associated trauma. Improved techniques in blood pressure management have decreased its incidence in the United States; however, once ICH occurs, there is still a high risk of morbidity and death. ICH management typically revolves around controlling size growth and supportive care while allowing the blood to reabsorb, though new techniques are being explored.

In this chapter, you will learn how to:

- Identify various causes of ICH.
- Utilize anticoagulant reversal agents.
- Implement neurosurgical interventions for ICH

EPIDEMIOLOGY

- Occurs in approximately 1 out of every 10,000 persons
- More common in African Americans and Asians
- Incidence increases with age
- More common in men than women
- More frequently occurs in low socioeconomic groups

PATHOPHYSIOLOGY

- Common causes (Table 6.1)
  - Hypertension related
    - Sixty percent of cases
    - Occurs when small arteriole ruptures
  - Cerebral amyloid angiopathy (CAA)
    - Results from amyloid deposits within vasculature
    - Typically lobar

RISK FACTORS

- Modifiable risk factors
  - Hypertension
  - Smoking

Table 6.1

Common Causes of ICH

AVM

Cavernoma
Arteriovenous malformation
Venous angioma
Capillary telangiectasis

Coagulopathies

Hereditary (von Willebrand's disease)
Medication-acquired (aspirin, heparin, warfarin, Plavix)
Disease-related (myeloproliferative and dysplastic disorders, uremia, liver
    disease, lupus, multiple myeloma)

Hypertension

Tumors

Glioblastoma
Melanoma
Renal cell carcinoma
Bronchogenic carcinoma

Vasculopathies

Cerebral amyloid angiopathy
Polyarteritis nodosa
Necrotizing vasculopathy
Moya moya
Vasculitis
Venous sinus thrombosis

AVM, arteriovenous malformation; ICH, intracerebral hemorrhage.

- Alcohol use
- Drug use
- Decreased low-density lipoprotein (LDL)
- Nonmodifiable risk factors
  - Age
  - Sex
  - CAA
  - Ethnicity
  - Race

CLINICAL MANIFESTATIONS

- Vary dependent upon bleed size and location (Table 6.2)
- Most common manifestations
  - Headache
  - Nausea
  - Vomiting

DIAGNOSTIC STUDIES

- Neuroimaging
  - Noncontrast CT scan
    - Complete as soon as possible
    - Shows ICH size and location
    - Identifies midline shift and/or hydrocephalus

Fast Facts

CT with contrast may demonstrate extravasation into the ICH known as "spot sign." This is predictive of increasing ICH volume.

  - MRI
    - Same benefit as above
    - Additionally can demonstrate vascular abnormalities, such as arteriovenous malformation (AVM)
    - May be able to identify age of hematoma
  - Angiography
    - Complete if concern for vascular abnormality

Table 6.2

Presentation of ICH Based Upon Location

Location	Important Facts	Motor	Sensory	Pupils	Eye Movement	Additional Features
Caudate nucleus with intraventricular extension	—	Contralateral hemiparesis (mild)	—	Constricted ipsilaterally	Conjugate deviation toward lesion; mild ptosis	Headache; meningismus; abulia
Putamen	Most common site for hypertensive ICH	Contralateral hemiparesis	Contralateral hemisensory loss	Normal to dilated on side of lesion dependent upon lesion size	Conjugate deviation toward lesion	Dominant lesions often have aphasia; decreased level of consciousness in large bleeds
Thalamus	—	Variable contralateral hemiparesis	Prominent contralateral hemisensory loss	Constricted; sluggishly reactive to light bilaterally	Restricted upward eye movement; eyes deviated downward and medially; retracted eyelids bilaterally	Dominant lesion aphasia; nondominant lesion neglect; early depressed level of consciousness; contralateral homonymous hemianopia if parietal–temporal involved

Occipital lobe	—	Transient, mild hemiparesis	Normal	Normal	Normal	Contralateral hemianopia
Pons	—	Quadriparesis; facial weakness	—	Constricted—pinpoint, but minimally reactive to light	Vertical eye movement intact; unable to move eyes horizontally	Early coma
Cerebellum	Neurosurgical emergency	Ipsilateral limb ataxia; no hemiparesis	—	Mild constriction on side of lesion	Mild deviation to opposite side; sixth cranial nerve palsy—impaired movement toward side of lesion	Gait ataxia; severe headache with nausea and vomiting

ICH, intracerebral hemorrhage.

- Laboratory investigations
  - Complete blood cell count
  - Prothrombin time (PT)
  - Partial thromboplastin time (PTT)
  - International normalized ratio (INR)

Fast Facts

Consider the use of thromboelastogram (TEG) to guide transfusions to correct coagulopathy.

CLASSIFICATION

- ICH score (Table 6.3)

Fast Facts

The tentorium is part of the dura mater, which separates the cerebellum from the occipital lobe. Therefore, infratentorial refers to the brainstem, cerebellum, and pons.

Table 6.3

Scoring Values for Use in Calculation of the ICH Score

Feature	Finding	Points
GCS score	3–4	2
	5–12	1
	13–15	0
Age	≥80 y	1
	<80 y	0
Location	Infratentorial	1
	Supratentorial	0
ICH volume (Figure 6.1)	≥30 mL	1
	<30 mL	0
Intraventricular blood	Yes	1
	No	0
ICH score		0–6 points

GCS, Glasgow Coma Scale; ICH, intracerebral hemorrhage.

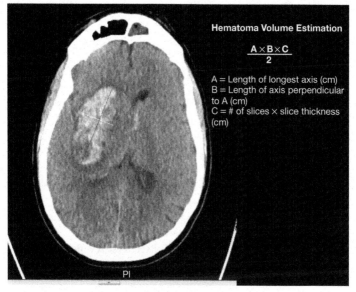

Figure 6.1 Calculating hematoma volume.
Note: Most centers utilize a slice thickness of 0.5 cm unless smaller slices are requested.

MANAGEMENT

- Supportive care
  - Blood pressure control
    - Goal systolic blood pressure (SBP) less than 140 mmHg
      - Antihypertensives

Fast Facts

Some guidelines allow for SBP up to 160 mmHg in patients with known hypertension.

- Intermittent
  - Labetalol 10 to 20 mg IV q15min
  - Hydralazine 10 to 20 mg IV q4h
- Continuous
  - Nicardipine infusion 5 to 15 mg/hr
  - Clevidipine infusion 1 to 21 mg/hr

- Reverse coagulopathy (Table 6.4)
  - Should be done as soon as possible
    - Three-factor prothrombin complex concentrate (PCC)
      - Factors II, IX, X, heparin
      - Bebulin
    - Four-factor PCC
      - Factors II, VII, IX, X, protein C/S, heparin, antithrombin III, albumin
      - Kcentra (Table 6.5)
    - Andexanet alfa
      - Not Food and Drug Administration (FDA) approved yet
      - Promising reversal agents for novel oral anticoagulant (NOAC) related bleeds
    - Vitamin K must be administered for reversal of warfarin-related coagulopathy

Fast Facts

Vitamin K administered intravenously is more effective than subcutaneous (SQ) vitamin K because of variable absorption when given subcutaneously. Intravenous (IV) vitamin K starts to act within 2 hours, whereas enteral vitamin K takes 6 hours or more.

  - Goal INR is typically less than 1.4

Fast Facts

Be aware of rebound coagulopathy that can occur after PCC administration for warfarin reversal, particularly if not administered with vitamin K. INR should be monitored every 6 hours for the first 24 hours and then daily for 3 to 5 days.

- Management of complications
  - Increased intracranial pressure (ICP)
  - Hydrocephalus

Table 6.4

Commonly Prescribed Anticoagulants With Their Reversal Agent	
Medication	Reversal
Warfarin	PCC + vitamin K
Heparin or low-molecular-weight heparin	Protamine
tPA	Cryoprecipitate ± antifibrinolytic agent, such as tranexamic acid
Dabigatran	Idarucizumab
Factor Xa inhibitors (Eliquis/Xarelto)	PCC
Antiplatelets	Withhold offending medication; *only if neurosurgical intervention planned,* consider platelets or desmopressin (DDAVP) if renal dysfunction present

PCC, prothrombin complex concentrate; tPA, tissue plasminogen activator.

Table 6.5

Recommended Kcentra Dosing Regimen for Prolonged INR in ICH		
INR	Kcentra Dose in Units of Factor IX/kg	Maximum Dose (Units)
2–3.9	25 ′ wt	2,500
4–6	35 ′ wt	3,500
>6	50 ′ wt	5,000

ICH, intracerebral hemorrhage; INR, international normalized ratio.

Fast Facts

Only a small percentage of patients with nontraumatic ICH have seizures; therefore prophylactic antiepileptic drugs are not recommended. However, there should be a low threshold to consider EEG in patients with persistent altered mental status inconsistent with ICH size and location.

- Neurosurgical intervention
  - Minimally invasive neurosurgery
    - Stereotactic endoscopic clot evacuation
      - Catheter placed within the clot and an aspirator is utilized to remove the hematoma
    - Fibrinolysis
      - Catheter placed within the clot and fibrinolytics administered to liquefy and drain the hematoma
  - Decompressive hemicraniectomy/craniotomy
    - Controversial—may or may not improve outcomes
    - Exception is patients with large cerebellar hemorrhage with brainstem compression—these patients benefit from early decompression

PROGNOSIS

- Forty percent case fatality at 1 month; 54% at 1 year

Fast Facts

Current guidelines advocate aggressive care for the first 24 hours to prevent a poor outcome becoming a self-fulfilling prophecy.

- Higher mortality rate in patients with anticoagulation-related ICH (Table 6.6)

Table 6.6

Thirty-Day Mortality Rate Based Upon ICH Score	
ICH Score	30-Day Mortality Rate (%)
0	0
1	13
2	26
3	72
4	97
5	100
6	100

ICH, intracerebral hemorrhage.

- Factors that affect prognosis:
  - Glasgow Coma Scale (GCS) score on arrival
  - ICH volume
  - Intraventricular extension
  - Location of bleed
  - Age
  - Chronic kidney disease
  - Nutritional status
  - Hyperglycemia

Bibliography

Anderson, C. S., Heeley, E., Huang, Y., Wang, J., Stapf, C., Delcourt, C., . . . Chalmers, J. (2013). Rapid blood-pressure lowering in patients with acute intracerebral hemorrhage. *The New England Journal of Medicine, 368*, 2355–2365. doi:10.1056/NEJMoa1214609

Firsching, R., Huber, M., & Frowein, R. A. (1991). Cerebellar haemorrhage: Management and prognosis. *Neurosurgical Review, 14*, 191–194. doi:10.1007/BF00310656

Hemphill, J. C. III, Greenberg, S. M., Anderson, C. S., Becker, K., Bendok, B. R., Cushman, M., . . . Woo, D. (2015). Guidelines for the management of spontaneous intracerebral hemorrhage: A guideline for healthcare professionals from the American Heart Association/American Stroke Association. *Stroke, 46*, 2032–2060. doi:10.1161/STR.0000000000000069

Hemphill, J. C., III, Bonovich, D. C., Besmertis, L., Manley, G. T., & Johnston, S. C. (2001). The ICH score: A simple, reliable grading scale for intracerebral hemorrhage. *Stroke, 32*, 891–897. doi:10.1161/01.STR.32.4.891

Kothari, R., Brott, T., Broderick, J., Barsan, W., Sauerbeck, L., Zuccarello, M., & Khoury, J. (1996). The ABCs of measuring intracerebral hemorrhage volumes. *Stroke, 27*, 1304–1305. doi:10.1161/01.STR.27.8.1304

7

Subarachnoid Hemorrhage

Subarachnoid hemorrhage (SAH) accounts for approximately 5% of strokes in the United States; however, it is associated with a high rate of morbidity and mortality. Data demonstrate that patients cared for by a neurocritical care specialist have improved outcomes compared to those cared for by a general intensivist. The understanding of the disease process and treatment strategies is useful to the neurocritical care provider. This chapter will focus on the background, diagnosis, and treatment of patients with SAH with most of the emphasis being specific to aneurysmal SAH.

In this chapter, you will learn how to:

- Identify the pathophysiology of SAH.
- Diagnose SAH.
- Analyze the complications of SAH and implement treatment strategies.

EPIDEMIOLOGY

The incidence of SAH does vary somewhat dependent upon region, with fewer reported cases in China and South America but an increased amount of cases in Finland and Japan. In the United States, the incidence is thought to be between 10 and 15 people per

Table 7.1

Risk Factors for SAH

Previous history of aneurysm or SAH

Family history of aneurysm or SAH

Hypertension

Smoking

Excessive alcohol consumption

Polycystic kidney disease

Marfan's syndrome

Ehler–Danlos syndrome, type 4

Coarctation of aorta

SAH, subarachnoid hemorrhage.

100,000, which is roughly 40,000 cases per year. Though SAH can occur at any age, the mean age of 55 years is younger than the average age of stroke in general. Aneurysmal SAH (aSAH) is more likely to occur in females. African Americans and Hispanic race are also associated with an increased incidence. Modifiable risk factors for aSAH include hypertension (HTN), alcohol and tobacco use, and cocaine use. Other risk factors are listed in Table 7.1.

Fast Facts

All first-degree relatives of someone with aSAH should be screened for aneurysms.

PATHOPHYSIOLOGY

SAH typically occurs as the result of aneurysmal rupture or trauma. Intracranial aneurysms are characterized by dilation of the arterial wall. Aneurysms typically occur as the result of structural changes of the arterial wall due to tissue degeneration or breakdown of the extracellular matrix, followed by smooth muscle cell apoptosis. These changes weaken the arterial wall, eventually causing it to dilate and balloon outward, forming an aneurysm. SAH occurs when the aneurysm then ruptures.

Anterior circulation aneurysms are more common than posterior. The anterior communicating artery is the most common location for intracranial aneurysm.

ANEURYSM TYPES

- Saccular
  - Berry
  - Most common (~90% of aneurysms)
  - Stereotypical ballooning; dome and neck connected to the more prominent vessel
  - Often found at arterial bifurcations
- Micro
  - Charcot–Bouchard aneurysms
  - Less than 2 mm in diameter
  - Most commonly caused by chronic HTN
  - Often found in basal ganglia microvessels
- Giant
  - Greater than 25 mm in diameter
  - So large that intact giant aneurysm can cause focal symptoms and intracranial HTN as a result of mass effect
- Fusiform
  - Dolichoectatic
  - Wide, thin segment of artery
  - Involve the entire circumference
  - Often found in vertebrobasilar system
  - Difficult to treat secondary to occlusion risk to perforating vessels
- Dissections
  - Pseudoaneurysms
  - Often affect vertebral arteries
  - Occur when there is rupture through the tunica adventitia
    - Causes SAH
    - Causes what appears to be pseudoaneurysms
- Mycotic
  - Rare
  - Infectious etiology
  - Often found in distal circulation

SIGNS AND SYMPTOMS

- Hallmark symptom is severe headache
  - Thunderclap
  - Often described as "worst headache of life"
  - Reaches maximum intensity within 30 to 60 seconds

The timing of headache maximum intensity is important to help differentiate between a patient with aSAH and a patient with daily migraines who may be having a very bad one.

- Sentinel headache
  - Patients often describe a warning headache preceding aSAH
  - Often occurs when there is a small aneurysmal leak
- Meningeal signs
  - Neck stiffness
  - Lower-back pain
  - Photophobia
- Nausea
- Vomiting
- Altered level of consciousness
  - Can range from sleepiness to comatose
- Seizures
  - In approximately 20% of patients
  - Prophylactic use of antiepileptic drugs (AEDs) is generally not recommended
  - AEDs should be used in patients with observed seizures
- May have focal symptoms based upon aneurysm location and mass effect

DIAGNOSIS

- Neuroimaging
  - Noncontrast head CT
    - Both sensitive and specific if performed within 6 hours
      - Sensitivity decreases over time
      - Generally not very sensitive after 1 week

- CT angiography (CTA)
  - Often done in conjunction with noncontrast CT
  - Able to detect aneurysms
  - May miss small or thrombosed aneurysms, particularly soon after bleeding occurs
- MRI
  - Better sensitivity than CT after 1 week
  - Does not require contrast for identification of aneurysms
  - Sensitive for blood when CT is indeterminate
    - Fluid-attenuated inversion recovery (FLAIR)
    - Proton density
    - Gradient echo
- Digital subtraction angiography (DSA)
  - Gold standard for aneurysm diagnosis
  - Performed in interventional radiology suite
  - Requires use of contrast agent to visualize cerebral arteries
  - Produces three-dimensional (3-D) real-time images
  - If initial DSA is negative, it should be repeated at neurosurgical team's preference
  - Risks
    - New ischemic stroke
    - Arterial perforation/dissection
    - Groin hematoma
    - Retroperitoneal hemorrhage
    - Kidney injury secondary to contrast agent
- Lumbar puncture (LP)
  - Can be performed at bedside or in interventional suite
  - Indication
    - CT negative with high suspicion for SAH
  - Most sensitive diagnostic test after 12 hours following symptom onset
  - It is important to measure the opening pressure during LP (elevated in two-thirds of patients with SAH)

Fast Facts

Two techniques can be used to differentiate between SAH and a traumatic LP. Xanthochromia (yellow tint that occurs as a result of red blood cell [RBC] breakdown) is *not* present in a traumatic LP. Also, CSF typically clears in a traumatic LP, whereas CSF remains bloody in acute SAH.

SCORING SCALES

- Hunt–Hess Scale (Table 7.2)
  - Describes initial clinical presentation
- World Federation of Neurosurgical Societies (WFNS) Scale (Table 7.3)
  - Describes initial clinical presentation
- Modified Fisher scale (Table 7.4)
  - Describes likelihood of vasospasm

Table 7.2

Using the Hunt–Hess Scale to Classify Severity of SAH

Grade	Description	Vasospasm Risk (%)
0	Unruptured aneurysm	0
1	Mild headache ± nuchal rigidity or no symptoms	22
2	Moderate-to-severe headache or nuchal rigidity; no neuro deficit except for CN palsy	33
3	Mild focal deficit; drowsiness or confusion	52
4	Stupor; moderate-to-severe hemiparesis	53
5	Coma; decerebrate posturing	74

CN, cranial nerve; SAH, subarachnoid hemorrhage.

Table 7.3

The WFNS Scale in Scoring SAH Severity

Grade	GCS Score	Motor Deficit	Survival Rate (%)
1	15	Absent	70
2	13–14	Absent	60
3	13–14	Present	50
4	7–12	Present or absent	40
5	3–6	Present or absent	10

GCS, Glasgow Coma Scale; SAH, subarachnoid hemorrhage; WFNS, World Federation of Neurosurgical Societies.

Table 7.4

The Modified Fisher Grading Scale in Scoring SAH Severity		
Grade	Description	Vasospasm (%)
1	Focal or diffuse thin SAH; no IVH	24
2	Focal or diffuse thin SAH; IVH	33
3	Thick SAH; no IVH	33
4	Thick SAH; IVH	40

Note: Thin SAH ≤1 mm depth; thick SAH ≥1 mm depth.
IVH, intraventricular hemorrhage; SAH, subarachnoid hemorrhage.

MEDICAL INTERVENTIONS

- Unsecured aneurysms
  - Initial management is geared toward avoiding rerupture
  - Serial neurological examinations
  - Pain management
    - Avoid straining or writhing as can cause aneurysmal rerupture
    - Utilize medications with short half-life
  - Blood pressure (BP) control
    - Well-accepted guideline is systolic blood pressure (SBP) goal less than 140 mmHg
    - Prevent hypotension as can cause secondary brain injury
    - Use short-acting, titratable medications for BP control
  - Achieve hemostasis
    - Goal international normalized ratio (INR) less than 1.4
    - Goal platelets greater than 50,000/µL
    - Antifibrinolytic agents may decrease re-rupture risk; however, they also may increase thrombotic complications
- Suggested dosing regimens of antifibrinolyric agents are as follows:
  - Aminocaproic acid 4 g IV g 1, followed by 1 g/hr for maximum of 72 hours or until aneurysm secured
  - Tranexamic acid 1 g IV g 1, followed by 1 g infusion over 8 hours
    - Reverse blood thinners if present
  - Nausea control
    - Use liberally if vomiting, as can lead to rerupture

NEUROSURGICAL INTERVENTIONS

- External ventricular drain (EVD)
  - Indications
    - Obstructive hydrocephalus
      - Thick blood from SAH prevents the free flow of cerebrospinal fluid (CSF) through the spinal canal
      - Decreases pressure and mass effect by way of CSF diversion
    - Increased intracranial pressure monitoring
      - Occurs as a result of hydrocephalus
      - Can progress to herniation syndrome if left untreated
- Lumbar drain
  - Alternative to EVD placement
  - Complimentary to EVD placement
    - May decrease patient discomfort/meningeal signs because promotes drainage of thick blood that has been pulled to the lumbar region by gravity
    - May decrease vasospasm incidence
  - Serial LPs or high-volume LP may be used instead of lumbar drain placement
- Surgical clipping
  - Requires open craniotomy
    - The neurosurgeon dissects to the artery where the aneurysm is located
    - A temporary clip is placed on the adjacent artery to diminish arterial blood flow and deflate the aneurysm
    - The neck of the aneurysm is secured with a titanium clip across the neck of the aneurysm
    - Risks
      - Increased risk of vasospasm
      - Cerebral ischemia
      - Bleeding
      - Infection
- Endovascular intervention
  - Minimally invasive
  - Can be performed on nonintubated patients utilizing conscious sedation alone
  - Malleable coils are placed within the body of the aneurysm and induce embolization of the aneurysm; this essentially seals the neck of the aneurysm and prevents further blood flow into the aneurysm
  - A newer endovascular intervention is stent placement to divert blood flow around the site of the aneurysm
  - Risks

- ❏ Prolonged radiation
- ❏ Vessel perforation
- ❏ Thromboembolism
- ❏ Acute ischemic stroke
- ❏ Dislodged coil
- ❏ Hematoma formation at arterial access site
- ❏ Retroperitoneal hemorrhage

COMPLICATIONS OF SAH

Vasospasm/delayed cerebral ischemia (DCI)
- Vasospasm
  - The narrowing of cerebral arteries that occurs after SAH
  - Typically occurs days 4 to 14, peaking days 7 to 10
  - Resolves by day 21
  - High incidence (between 70% and 90%)
  - Often asymptomatic
  - Does not always require intervention

Fast Facts

When vasospasm occurs with clinical deterioration, it is a medical emergency and requires prompt treatment.

- DCI
  - Delayed cerebral infarction
  - Characterized by any new neurological deficit related to ischemia
  - Typically lasts greater than 1 hour
  - Second-most common cause of morbidity and death following initial aneurysm rupture

Fast Facts

There is no correlation between aneurysm location and the vessel associated with vasospasm or DCI.

- Signs and symptoms
  - Any change in mental status should be investigated as potentially vasospasm/DCI, including the following:

- New-onset delirium
- Lethargy
- Headache
- Focal changes
- Diagnosis
  - Neuroimaging
    - Transcranial Doppler (TCD)
      - Often performed serially
      - More screening than truly diagnostic
      - Increased velocities indicate vasospasm
    - Magnetic resonance angiography (MRA) or CTA
      - CT perfusion may be more accurate in predicting need for endovascular intervention
    - DSA
      - Gold standard for vasospasm diagnosis
      - One hundred percent sensitivity and specificity for vasospasm detection
      - Same risks as described in endovascular intervention
      - Cannot identify ischemic areas
      - Can intervene at the same time as diagnosis
- Medical interventions
  - Nimodipine
    - Does not reduce vasospasm or risk of developing vasospasm
    - Does reduce risk of DCI
    - Recommended 21-day course
    - Hypotension is common side effect and should be avoided

Fast Facts

Nimodipine can be given more frequently at a decreased dosage in patients who experience hypotension as a side effect.

  - Blood pressure management
    - Liberalize BP versus induced HTN
  - Volume management
    - Goal: euvolemia
    - Can be challenging if polyuria occurs
      - Polyuria should be investigated and diagnosed so that it may be treated appropriately (Table 7.5)
    - No benefit to hypervolemia; actually worsens outcomes

Table 7.5

Interpreting Common Urine Abnormalities That May Occur in SAH

	Serum Na	Urine Na	Serum Osmolality	Urine Osmolality	Volume Status	Urine Output	Treatment
CSW	Decreased	>20 mmol/L	Decreased	Normal	Hypovolemic	Increased	Volume replacement, Na supplementation, ± fludrocortisone (Florinef)
SIADH	Decreased	>40 mmol/L	Decreased	Increased (>300 mmol/kg)	Euvolemic	Decreased	Fluid restriction may not be appropriate if in SAH; hypertonic (3%) saline infusion
DI	Increased	<20 mmol/L	Increased (>300 mmol/kg)	Decreased (<300 mmol/kg)	Euvolemic or hypovolemic	Increased	Volume replacement; desmopressin (DDAVP)

CSW, cerebral salt wasting; DI, diabetes insipidus; SAH, subarachnoid hemorrhage; SIADH, syndrome of inappropriate diuretic hormone secretion.

- Neurosurgical interventions
  - Intra-arterial vasodilators
  - Intraventricular vasodilators
  - Balloon angioplasty

Bibliography

Connolly, E. S. Jr, Rabinstein, A. A., Carhuapoma, J. R., Derdeyn, C. P., Dion, J., Higashida, R. T., . . . Vespa, P. (2012). Guidelines for the management of aneurysmal subarachnoid hemorrhage: A guideline for healthcare professionals from the American Heart Association/American Stroke Association. *Stroke, 43,* 1711–1737. doi:10.1161/STR.0b013e3182587839

Diringer, M. N., Bleck, T. P., Claude Hemphill, J., III, Menon, D., Shutter, L., Vespa, P., . . . Zipfel, G. (2011). Critical care management of patients following aneurysmal subarachnoid hemorrhage: Recommendations from the Neurocritical Care Society's Multidisciplinary Consensus Conference. *Neurocritical Care, 15,* 211–240. doi:10.1007/s12028-011-9605-9

Hillman, J., Fridriksson, S., Nilsson, O., Yu, Z., Säveland, H., & Jakobsson, K.-E. (2002). Immediate administration of tranexamic acid and reduced incidence of early rebleeding after aneurysmal subarachnoid hemorrhage: A prospective randomized study. *Journal of Neurosurgery, 97,* 771–778. doi:10.3171/jns.2002.97.4.0771

III

Trauma

8

Traumatic Brain Injury

Traumatic brain injury (TBI) refers to neurological insult that occurs as a result of trauma. This can occur from many mechanisms but is commonly associated with motor vehicle accidents, blunt trauma, or falls, among many others. This chapter will briefly describe the epidemiology and classification of TBI overall, followed by a more in-depth look at three common types of TBI.

In this chapter, you will learn how to:

- Differentiate between epidural and subdural hematoma (SDH) on imaging.
- Describe management priorities in a patient with TBI.
- Prognosticate a patient with severe diffuse axonal injury (DAI).

EPIDEMIOLOGY

- Incidence
  - United States
    - People annually diagnosed with TBI: 1.7 million
      - Seventy-five percent of patients have mild forms of TBI
- Male greater than female
- Frequently occurs in children 0 to 14 years
  - Most common cause of death in young adults in developed countries

CLASSIFICATION

- Glasgow Coma Scale (GCS) system
  - Mild: GCS score 13 to 15
  - Moderate: GCS score 9 to 12
  - Severe: GCS score 3 to 8

Fast Facts

Most classification systems specify that the score should be performed within 48 hours from presentation but after resuscitation.

- Marshall classification
  - Diffuse injury I: No pathology visible on CT
  - Diffuse injury II: Cisterns present with 0 to 5 mm midline shift ± lesion densities present; no lesion greater than 25 cm³
  - Diffuse injury III: Compression of cisterns, may be visibly absent, midline shift 0 to 5 mm; no lesion greater than 25 cm³
  - Diffuse injury IV: Midline shift greater than 5 mm; no lesion greater than 25 cm³
  - Evacuated mass lesion V: Any surgically evacuated lesion
  - Nonevacuated mass lesion VI: Lesion greater than 25 cm³; not surgically evacuated
- Mayo Classification System for Traumatic Brain Injury Severity
  - Moderate to severe
    - Criteria
      - Death
      - Loss of consciousness 30+ minutes
      - Posttraumatic amnesia (PTA) of 24+ hours
      - Worst GCS score in first 24 hours less than 13 not due to sedation/intoxication
      - Evidence of hematoma, hemorrhage, or contusion
  - Mild
    - Criteria
      - Loss of consciousness less than 30 minutes
      - PTA less than 24 hours
      - Depressed, basilar, or linear skull fracture
  - Possible TBI
    - Criteria
      - One or more of the following symptoms after trauma

- Blurred vision
- Confusion
- Dizziness
- Feeling "dazed"
- Headache
- Nausea

EPIDURAL HEMATOMA

- Definition
  - Blood collection between the dura and skull (Figure 8.1)
- Epidemiology
  - Uncommon
  - Incidence between 1% and 4% in trauma
    - Higher incidence in autopsy
  - Most common in adolescents and young adults
    - Mean age 20 to 30 years
    - Rare after the age of 50 years
  - Predominance in trauma; rarely nontraumatic etiology
- Pathophysiology
  - Lateral acceleration force along the skull produces injury to vasculature or brain parenchyma, resulting in hematoma

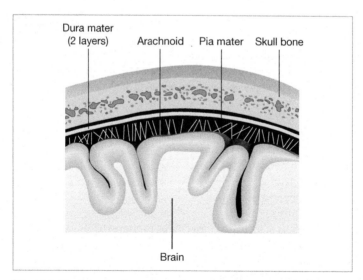

Figure 8.1 Meninges layers.
Source: Morrison, K. (2018). *Fast facts for stroke care nursing: An expert care guide* (2nd ed., p. 13). New York, NY: Springer Publishing.

- Most commonly caused by middle meningeal artery tearing
  - Results in epidural hematoma (EDH) in middle cranial fossa over the cerebral convexity
- Can also occur with anterior meningeal artery rupture
  - EDH then found in anterior cranial fossa
- Rarely due to dural arteriovenous fistula (dAVF)
  - At vertex

Fast Facts

Approximately 15% of EDHs are a result of venous bleeding.

- Often co-exists with skull fractures
- Presentation
  - Can be variable dependent upon size and location of hematoma
  - Common presentation
    - Lucid interval
      - Initial loss of consciousness, followed by interval recovery, and then deterioration over hours

Fast Facts

If EDH is caused by arterial tearing, it can progress rapidly, which is why EDH is considered a medical emergency. EDH resultant from venous bleeding presents with slower neurological deterioration.

- Headache
- Altered mental status
- Vomiting
- Seizures
- Hemiparesis
- Drowsiness
- Signs of increased intracranial pressure (ICP)
  - Ipsilateral dilated pupil
  - Cushing reflex
    - Hypertension
    - Bradycardia
    - Respiration depression

- Diagnostic evaluation
  - Neuroimaging
    - Noncontrast CT of head
      - Lens-shaped or biconvex blood pattern
      - May not be present on initial CT in almost 1 out of 10 patients
        - Causes of EDH might not appear
          - Anemia
          - Shock
          - Slow venous bleed

Fast Facts

EDH's lens-shaped appearance is due to its inability to cross sutural margins; however, it does cross the dural attachments.

    - MRI
      - Can be used when strong suspicion of EDH exists without evidence on CT (Table 8.1)
      - More sensitive, particularly at vertex
    - Angiography
      - For strong suspicion of dAVF
      - Diagnose vascular lesion
  - Laboratory investigations
    - Complete blood cell count
    - Prothrombin time (PT)/international normalized ratio (INR) and partial thromboplastin time (PTT)

Table 8.1

MRI Findings Present in Epidural Hematoma

Time	MRI Findings	Cause
Acute	Hypointense on T2	Deoxyhemoglobin presence
Following weeks	Hyperintense on T1 and T2	Degradation of deoxyhemoglobin to methemoglobin
Following months	Hypointense on T1	Only hemosiderin exists

- Management
  - Supportive care
    - Airway
    - Blood pressure management
      - Avoid hypertension to prevent hematoma expansion
      - Avoid hypotension/shock to ensure adequate cerebral perfusion pressure (CPP)
    - Neurosurveillance
      - Serial CT scans are indicated if surgery is not pursued
  - Medication
    - Reversal of anticoagulation
      - Please see Chapter 6 for recommendations for reversal of anticoagulants
    - Blood pressure control
    - Osmotic agents
      - If evidence of increased ICP
  - Neurosurgical intervention

Fast Facts

Most patients with EDH and neurological deficits on exam will require emergent surgery for evacuation of hematoma.

  - Craniotomy
    - Hematoma evacuation
    - Ligation of bleeding vessel
  - Burr hole
    - Relieves intracranial pressure
    - Emergency treatment
    - Consider if specialized neurosurgeons are not available
  - Indications for surgery
    - Hematoma size greater than 30 cm^3
    - GCS score less than 9 and anisocoria

Fast Facts

Patients who undergo early neurosurgical intervention typically have better outcomes than patients who have delayed intervention.

- Prognosis
  - Mortality
    - Approximately 10%
    - Predictors of good outcome
      - GCS score 8 or more at admission
      - Patients who undergo hematoma evacuation
    - Predictors of poor outcome
      - Low GCS score
      - Pupil abnormalities
      - Older age
      - Elevated ICP after hematoma evacuation
      - Time between deterioration and surgery
      - Hematoma volume greater than 30 cm^3
      - Midline shift greater than 1 cm

SUBDURAL HEMATOMA

- Definition
  - Blood between the arachnoid membrane and the dura
- Epidemiology
  - Incidence is increasing
  - Approximately 40 cases per 100,000 persons
  - Most common cause is head trauma
    - Motor vehicle accidents
    - Falls
    - Assault
  - Highest incidence of acute traumatic SDH is in middle-aged men
  - Overall highest incidence in elderly
  - Risk factors
    - Cerebral atrophy
      - Elderly
      - TBI
    - Antithrombotic use
- Pathophysiology
  - Lateral acceleration force along the skull produces injury to vasculature or brain parenchyma, resulting in hematoma
  - Most commonly caused by tears to the veins that drain the surface of the brain to the dural sinuses
    - Most commonly located in frontoparietal region

Table 8.2

Classification of SDH by Time and CT Appearance

	Time	CT Appearance
Acute	1–2 d	Hyperdense
Subacute	3–14 d	Iso- or hypodense
Chronic	15+ d	Iso- or hypodense

SDH, subdural hematoma.

- ■ Can also be caused by arterial rupture
  - ❑ Most commonly located in temporoparietal region
- ■ Presentation
  - ■ Can be variable dependent upon size and location of hematoma
  - ■ Common presentations
    - ❑ Coma
      - ● Fifty percent of cases
    - ❑ Lucid interval
    - ❑ Otherwise similar presentation to EDH
- ■ Diagnostic evaluation
  - ■ Neuroimaging
    - ❑ Noncontrast CT of head
      - ● Crescent-shaped blood pattern

Fast Facts

SDH's crescent-shaped appearance is due to its ability to cross sutural margins but not dural attachments.

- ● Density of blood products can help differentiate between time of bleeding (Table 8.2)
- ● SDH greater than 5 mm is easily identified; SDH less than 3 mm is often missed on the initial scan
- ❑ MRI
  - ● More sensitive in the identification of small SDH
- ■ Laboratory investigations
  - ❑ Complete blood cell count
  - ❑ PT/INR and PTT

- Management
  - Supportive care
    - Airway
    - Blood pressure management
      - Avoid hypertension to prevent hematoma expansion
      - Avoid hypotension/shock to ensure adequate CPP
    - Neurosurveillance
      - Serial CT scans are indicated if surgery is not pursued
  - Medication
    - Reversal of anticoagulation
      - Please see Chapter 6 for recommendations for reversal of anticoagulants
    - Blood pressure control
    - Osmotic agents
      - If evidence of increased ICP
  - Neurosurgical intervention
    - Craniotomy
      - Hematoma evacuation
      - Ligation of bleeding vessel
    - Burr hole
      - Relieves intracranial pressure
      - Emergency treatment
    - Decompressive craniectomy
    - Indications for surgery
      - Neurological deterioration with recovery potential
      - Clot thickness greater than 1 cm
      - Midline shift greater than 5 mm
      - Anisocoria
      - Evidence of increased ICP or herniation syndromes
- Prognosis
  - Mortality
    - Fifty percent in patients with acute SDH who require surgical intervention
    - Recurrence
      - Rare in acute SDH
      - More common (~30%) in chronic SDH

DIFFUSE AXONAL INJURY

- Epidemiology
  - Higher incidence of DAI with severe TBI
  - Commonly associated high-speed motor-vehicle accidents

- Pathophysiology
  - Occurs as a result of shearing to white matter tracts of the brain
    - Typically the result of acceleration/deceleration forces
  - This shearing motion also damages brain axons at the gray–white matter junction
    - Subsequently, the interconnection of neurons is disrupted, which in turn affects brain functioning
  - Followed by cell damage and edema
  - Corpus callosum and brainstem are commonly affected
- Classification
  - The Adams Diffuse Axonal Injury Grading
    - Grade 1: Mild
      - Microscopic white matter changes in cerebral cortex, corpus callosum, and brainstem
    - Grade 2: Moderate
      - Gross focal lesions in corpus callosum
    - Grade 3: Severe
      - Gross focal lesions in corpus callosum and brainstem
- Presentation
  - Varies dependent upon grade
  - Grade 1: Mild
    - Vague symptoms
    - Headache
    - Dizziness
    - Nausea/vomiting
    - Fatigue

Fast Facts

It is believed that concussion may be a form of mild DAI.

  - Grade 2 to 3: Moderate to severe
    - Symptoms remain vague
    - Altered level of consciousness
    - Coma
- Diagnosis
  - Clinical diagnosis can be made when there is persistent GCS score less than 8 for more than 6 hours following TBI
  - Neuroimaging

- ❏ CT
  - Difficult to diagnose from CT
  - May be normal
- ❏ MRI
  - More sensitive than CT
    - ○ Sensitivity declines over time
  - Susceptibility-weighted imaging (SWI) and gradient recalled echo (GRE) sequences
    - ○ More sensitive to paramagnetic blood
  - Nonhemorrhagic lesions better seen on fluid-attenuated inversion recovery (FLAIR)

Fast Facts

The absence of lesions on CT or MRI does not exclude the diagnosis of DAI.

- ■ Management
  - ▪ Supportive care
    - ❏ Airway
      - Intubation
    - ❏ Breathing
      - Avoidance of hypoxia
      - Consideration of use of hyperventilation (goal CO_2 30–35 mmHg) to transiently decrease ICP

Fast Facts

Hypoxia and hypotension in DAI are associated with increased mortality and should be avoided at all costs.

- ❏ Circulation
  - Avoid hypotension
    - ○ Hypotension decreases cerebral perfusion
- ❏ ICP
  - Monitoring
    - ○ Indicated in GCS score less than 8
    - ○ Limited exam due to other injuries or medication
  - Prompt treatment of increased ICP

- Medication
  - Osmotic agents for increased ICP
  - Antiepileptic agents
    - Prophylactic
      - Seven-day course
- Neurosurgical intervention
  - ICP monitor placement
- Prognosis
  - Clinical status persists for 2+ years
  - Poor prognosis for patients with severe DAI
  - Most common cause of morbidity and death following TBI
  - Most common cause of coma, disability, and persistent vegetative state following TBI
  - Number of identifiable lesions on imaging correlates with patient outcome

Bibliography

Carney, N., Totten, A. M., O'Reilly, C., Ullman, J. S., Hawryluk, G. W., Bell, M. J., . . . Ghajar, J. (2016). Guidelines for the management of severe traumatic brain injury, fourth edition. *Neurosurgery, 80*, 6–15. doi:10.1227/NEU.0000000000001432

Coronado, V. G., McGuire, L., Faul, M., Sugarman, D. E., & Pearson, W. S. (2013). Traumatic brain injury epidemiology and public health issues. In N. D. Zasler, D. I. Katz, R. D. Zafonte, D. B. Arciniegas, M. R. Bullock, & J. S. Kreutzer (Eds.), *Brain injury medicine: Principles and practice* (2nd ed., pp. 84–100). New York, NY: Demos Medical.

Malec, J. F., Brown, A. W., Leibson, C. L., Flaada, J. T., Mandrekar, J. N., Diehl, N. N., & Perkins, P. K. (2007). The Mayo classification system for traumatic brain injury severity. *Journal of Neurotrauma, 24*(9), 1417–1424. doi:10.1089/neu.2006.0245

Marshall, L. F., Marshall, S. B., Klauber, M. R., van Berkum Clark, M., Eisenberg, H. M., Jane, J. A., . . . Foulkes, M. A. (1991). A new classification of head injury based on computerized tomography. *Journal of Neurosurgery, 75*, S14–S20. Retrieved from http://thejns.org/doi/pdf/10.3171/sup.1991.75.1s.0s14

Morrison, K. (2018). *Fast facts for stroke care nursing: An expert care guide* (2nd ed.). New York, NY: Springer Publishing.

Viera, R. C., Wellingson, S. V., de Oliveira, D. V., Teixeira, M. J., de Andrade, A. F., & Sousa, R. M. (2016). Diffuse axonal injury: Epidemiology, outcome and associated risk factors. *Frontiers in Neurology, 7*, 179. doi:10.3389/fneur.2016.00178

9

Spinal Cord Injury

Acute spinal cord injury (SCI) can be a neurological emergency. As a result of improved safety measures, such as seat belts and improved neurosurgical care, the prevalence of complete cord lesions has decreased. Though trauma is a frequent cause of SCI, it may occur for many reasons and the type and degree of injury can be highly variable. This chapter will describe acute SCI.

In this chapter, you will learn how to:

- Review spinal cord anatomy and injury.
- Document neurological exam findings.
- Manage SCI and its complications.

EPIDEMIOLOGY

- Incidence
  - Varies dependent upon region of the world
  - United States
    - Ten thousand people are diagnosed with acute SCI each year
- Male greater than female (4:1)
- Bimodal distribution
  - Peaks
    - Early adults associated with motor vehicle accidents
    - Elderly associated with falls
  - Median age 37 years
- Trauma is the most common cause

- Location of SCI
  - Cervical spine most common
    - Fifty to seventy-five percent of SCI
  - Thoracic
    - Fifteen to thirty percent
  - Lumbosacral
    - Ten to twenty percent

PATHOPHYSIOLOGY

- Two stages that occur sequentially
  - Stage I
    - Immediate compression applied to spinal cord at time of injury
    - Resultant
      - Petechial hemorrhage of the gray/white matter
      - Axonal severing
      - Focal tissue destruction
  - Stage II
    - Secondary injury extends initial injury and continues for weeks
    - Resultant
      - Edema
      - Decreased spinal cord blood flow
        - Resultant infarction
      - Glial scar formation
        - Prevents axonal tract regeneration

REVIEW OF SPINAL ANATOMY

- Spine has three distinct columns
  - Anterior column
    - Contents
      - Anterior longitudinal ligament
      - Anterior half of vertebral body, disc, and annulus
  - Middle column
    - Contents
      - Posterior half of vertebral body, disc, and annulus
      - Posterior longitudinal ligament
  - Posterior column
    - Contents
      - Facet joints

- Ligamentum flavum
- Posterior elements
- Interconnecting ligaments

TERMINOLOGY

- Radiculopathy
  - Nerve root compression
- Myelopathy
  - Spinal cord compression
- Myeloradiculopathy
  - Compression of both the spinal cord and nerve root

CLINICAL PRESENTATION

- Variable presentation dependent upon cause of SCI
  - Common presenting symptoms
    - Pain
    - Weakness
    - Altered sensation
    - Urinary retention/incontinence
  - Some well-known spinal cord syndromes have specific exam findings (Table 9.1)
- History
  - Mechanism of injury (trauma)

Table 9.1

	Anterior Cord Syndrome	Brown–Séquard Syndrome	Central Cord Syndrome
Common Spinal Cord Syndromes With Etiology and Motor–Sensory Description			
Etiology	Ischemic injury or anterior disc herniation	Partial cord transection	Central spinal cord lesion
Motor	Complete loss of function	Hemiparesis	Weakness: greater in upper extremities than lower extremities
Sensory	Impaired below level of lesion with preserved function of the posterior column	Ipsilateral proprioception loss, contralateral loss of pain and temperature sensation	Decreased pain and temperature sensation over the arms, "cape-like" distribution

- Timetable for development of symptoms is important
- Fluctuating symptoms may occur

PHYSICAL ASSESSMENT

Fast Facts

All exams should be performed utilizing the International Standards for Neurological Classification of Spinal Cord Injury (ISNCSCI) to standardize the approach to acute SCI patients (see Appendix B: ISNCSCI Worksheet).

- Neurological examination
  - Motor
    - All muscle groups should be graded
    - 0 (total paralysis) to 5 (normal)
    - Some muscle groups localize to specific areas of the spine (Table 9.2)
  - Sensory
    - Thorough sensory exam includes
      - Pinprick
      - Vibration
      - Position
      - Touch
        - Light
        - Pressure
      - Temperature

Table 9.2

Level of Spinal Cord Injury and Affected Muscle Group	
Muscle Group	**Where Localizes to Spine**
Arm abduction	C5
Forearm extension	C5
Forearm flexion	C5, C6
Knee extension	L3, L4
Foot and great toe dorsiflexion	L5
Plantar flexion	S1

The exam at 72 hours is often considered the "baseline" exam and is used for comparison during follow-ups.

- Pain
  - Spine pain is often characterized as sharp and stabbing
- Tone
  - Examination of muscles' resistance to passive motion
  - May distinguish between upper and lower motor neuron disorder
- Determine level of spine involved
  - Level of normal motor and sensory function bilaterally
- Determine degree of injury
  - Grade
    - Complete loss involves both motor and sensory
    - Incomplete
  - Stability
    - Stable
      - Only anterior column affected
    - Unstable
      - Anterior and middle column involvement
      - All three columns

In multiple sclerosis, sensory symptoms are often the presenting symptoms, whereas motor or sphincter dysfunction is the most common presenting symptom in other causes.

DIAGNOSTICS

- Neuroimaging

The first priority of neuroimaging is to identify if the patient has an unstable cervical/thoracic spine fracture or spine compression to facilitate early intervention.

- ▪ Radiograph
  - ❑ Anteroposterior (AP) and lateral cervical plain film
    - ● Advanced trauma life support (ATLS) protocol
    - ● Identifies overt fractures
    - ● Omit if CT obtained
  - ❑ Plain spine films
    - ● Serial films
- ▪ CT
  - ❑ Identify fracture and dislocations
  - ❑ CT myelography can be used in patients who cannot undergo MRI

Fast Facts

All patients with acute trauma and altered mental status should undergo CT of the cervical spine.

- ▪ MRI
  - ❑ Better demonstrates soft tissue, including
    - ● Spinal cord
    - ● Nerve roots
    - ● Intervertebral discs
  - ❑ Best to obtain measurements of spinal cord compression
    - ● Maximum spinal cord compression (MSCC)
    - ● Maximum canal compromise (MCC)

MANAGEMENT

- ■ Medical management
  - ▪ Pulmonary
    - ❑ Low threshold for intubation
      - ● Particularly for cervical spine injury
      - ● Lesions above C4 often have shortness of breath and increased work of breathing and air hunger
      - ● Lesions above C3 have diaphragmatic weakness and require intubation
      - ● Lower lesions may also ultimately require ventilator support if the patient is unable to adequately cough
  - ▪ Cardiac support
    - ❑ Autonomic instability can occur

- ❏ Bradycardia is common
  - Atropine
  - Temporary pacemaker
- ❏ Hypotension is common
  - All potential causes of shock should be investigated prior to an assumption that hypotension is related to SCI
    - ○ Hypovolemic or hemorrhagic shock is a more common cause of hypotension after trauma than neurogenic shock
  - Spinal shock refers to loss of spinal reflex activity below the level of SCI
  - Neurogenic shock refers to loss of sympathetic outflow
    - ○ Vasoplegia and bradycardia occur
    - ○ Low systemic vascular resistance (SVR)
    - ○ Warm shock
  - Blood pressure (BP) support
    - ○ Volume resuscitation first
    - ○ Vasopressors may be necessary after euvolemia is established
      - – Norepinephrine
      - – Epinephrine
      - – Dopamine

Fast Facts

Goal mean arterial pressure (MAP) for a patient with SCI is greater than 85 mmHg or systolic blood pressure (SBP) greater than 120 mmHg to prevent cord ischemia.

- ▪ Prophylaxis
  - ❏ High risk of venous thromboembolism
    - Pneumatic compression devices
    - Early pharmacologic prophylaxis
      - ○ Unfractionated heparin
      - ○ Low-molecular-weight heparin
    - If contraindicated or delayed, consideration of inferior vena cava filter
- ▪ Temperature
  - ❏ Hyperthermia common early on
    - Strive for normothermia
    - Hyperthermia associated with worse neurological outcomes

- ❏ Poikilothermia can occur later on
- ▪ Elimination
  - ❏ Urinary retention and constipation may occur
  - ❏ The patient also may have incontinence of urine/stool
  - ❏ Hypervigilance to avoid infection and skin breakdown
- ▪ Pharmacologic management
  - ▪ Steroids
    - ❏ Controversial
    - ❏ No longer standard of care
    - ❏ May have slightly improved motor function if given early
    - ❏ Associated with more complications, particularly infectious
- ▪ Neurosurgical interventions
  - ▪ Urgent neurosurgical evaluation
    - ❏ Spinal cord decompression and stabilization
      - Indications
        - ○ Cord compression with accompanying neurological deficit
        - ○ Unstable vertebral fractures
      - Improved outcomes when completed within 24 hours

PROGNOSIS

- ▪ Prognosis varies widely dependent upon the type and severity of injury
- ▪ Patients without spinal cord signal change on MRI typically have better recovery potential
- ▪ Hematomas within the spinal cord or spinal cord transection typically have higher risk for morbidity/mortality

Bibliography

Consortium for Spinal Cord Medicine. (2008). *Early acute manage-ment in adults with spinal cord injury: A clinical practice guideline for health-care professionals.* Washington, DC: Paralyzed Veterans of America. Retrieved from https://www.pva.org/CMSPages/GetFile.aspx?guid=57fa58f9-e3b6-4be3-ad36-c6c5da5caa35

Licina, P., & Nowitzke, A. M. (2005). Approach and considerations regarding the patient with spinal injury. *Injury, 36*(Suppl. 2), B2–B12. doi:10.1016/j.injury.2005.06.010

Lindsey, R., Gugala, Z., & Pneumaticos, S. (2008). Injury to the vertebrae and spinal cord. In D. V. Feliciano, K. L. Mattox, & E. E. Moore (Eds.), *Trauma* (6th ed., pp. 479–510). New York, NY: McGraw-Hill.

IV

Neuromuscular Disorders

10

Guillain–Barré Syndrome

Guillain–Barré syndrome (GBS) is an autoimmune disorder of the peripheral nervous system. In GBS, the body's immune system destroys the myelin sheath and the body's ability to carry nerve signals, resulting in progressive weakness and possible autonomic dysfunction. This can create hemodynamic instability, requiring critical care interventions.

In this chapter, you will learn how to:

- Describe symptoms of GBS.
- Diagnose GBS.
- Review treatment strategies for GBS.

EPIDEMIOLOGY

- Rare: 1 to 2 in 100,000 per year
- Slightly more common in men than women (1.25:1)
- Bimodal incidence
  - Children and young adults
  - Patients over the age of 55 years
    - Higher rates in older adults
- Occurs more commonly during winter months

PATHOPHYSIOLOGY

The exact pathophysiology of GBS is poorly understood; however, it is typically agreed upon that the immune system is activated by some type of precipitating event/factor that leads to autoantibody production. Often, it appears that viral or bacterial infection occurs prior to GBS. One theory regarding the disease process is that the infection itself changes nervous system cells in a way that essentially makes them unrecognizable to the immune system, which subsequently treats them as foreign cells. Another theory is that the infection makes the immune system hyperactive and attacks the myelin.

In GBS, the peripheral nervous system is affected, mostly the spinal and cranial nerve roots; however, autonomic nerves can also be affected. Once the myelin sheath, which surrounds axons, or even axons themselves are destroyed by the immune system, the nerves cannot transmit signals appropriately. Because the nerve pathway between the brain and sensory is damaged, the brain cannot receive signals such as temperature, pain, or even the ability to feel texture. In order for recovery to occur, the immune response must be dampened to allow for nerve repair.

CLASSIFICATIONS

- Two main types
    - Acute inflammatory demyelinating polyneuropathy (AIDP)
        - In AIDP, the myelin sheath and Schwann-cell components are attacked
        - Most common form
    - Acute motor axonal neuropathy (AMAN)
        - In AMAN, the membranes of the nerve axon are attacked
        - Less common, more severe course of illness with slow recovery

CLINICAL COURSE

- Stage 1: Immune activation/prodromal (Figure 10.1)
    - Two-thirds of patients have preceding respiratory or gastrointestinal (GI) infection
    - Common pathogens are *Campylobacter*, *Mycoplasma*, or viruses
    - Typically prodromal illness occurs about 2 weeks prior to presentation

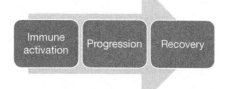

Figure 10.1 Disease course and stages of GBS.
GBS, Guillain–Barré syndrome.

- Stage 2: Progression
  - Week 1 to 2: Sensory and/or cranial nerve involvement
  - Peak clinical deficits typically occur at 2 weeks
  - Subacute GBS can progress up to 6 weeks
- Plateau stage: follows progression

Fast Facts

Despite initial improvement, 10% of patients deteriorate again and may benefit from another round of treatment.

- Stage 3: Recovery
  - Lasts months to years

SIGNS AND SYMPTOMS

- Weakness
  - Characterized as follows
    - Progressive
    - Bilateral
    - Symmetric
  - Most often starts in legs
  - Commonly ascending

Fast Facts

Variants to the typical presentation exist. Miller Fisher variant often presents as ophthalmoplegia, ataxia, and areflexia, which may then progress to limb weakness.

- Sensory involvement is common
  - Pain
    - Often described as in the low back or legs
    - Occurs prior to weakness in one third of cases
  - Paresthesias
    - Initial symptom in half of patients, eventually occurs in 70% to 90%
    - Occur distally first
  - Sensory loss often in patches
  - Fifteen percent of GBS patients have purely motor symptoms
- Cranial nerve VII
  - Symmetric: Early occurrence, parallel with weakness
  - Asymmetric: Later occurrence, other weakness may be improving
- Deep tendon reflex (DTR) loss
  - Areflexia occurs early in most patients (70%) but *can* occur late
  - Initially may be normal or hyperreflexic
  - Ankles most often lost
  - Biceps most often spared
  - If no loss of any DTR during disease course, consider other differential diagnoses
- Autonomic dysfunction
  - Occurs ~60% of the time
  - More common in severe syndrome

Fast Facts

Test autonomic function by applying bilateral ocular pressure for 25 seconds. If present, this will cause temporary bradycardia.

  - Blood pressure
    - Transient hyper- or hypotension
    - Orthostatic hypotension
    - More sensitive to antihypertensives
  - Cardiac arrhythmias
    - Tachycardia or bradycardia can occur
    - Dysrhythmias can occur
  - Bladder
    - Urinary retention
    - Sphincter symptoms in one tenth of patients

Table 10.1

Some Widely Accepted Criteria to Admit a Patient with GBS to ICU

Vital capacity <20 mL/kg

NIF <20 cm H_2O

Weak neck flexors, drooling, inability to control oral secretions

Airway protection concern

Need for mechanical ventilation

Rapid clinical progression

Pulmonary infiltrates

GBS, Guillain–Barré syndrome; NIF, negative inspiratory force.

- GI
  - Ileus
  - Diarrhea
  - Emesis
  - Abdominal pain
- Decreased sweating, salivation, and lacrimation
- Corneal ulcerations
- Respiratory failure (20–30% of cases; Table 10.1)

DIAGNOSIS

- Often based upon clinical pattern
- Cerebrospinal fluid (CSF)
  - Elevated protein without increased white blood cells (WBCs)
    - Greater than 0.55 g/L
    - Also referred to as "cytoalbuminological dissociation"
    - Only after 5 to 7 days of the disease
    - Absence does not rule out GBS
  - Some patients have oligoclonal banding
  - Five percent of patients have small increase in CSF cell count
- Blood tests
  - High immunoglobulin G (IgG)
  - Axonal forms of GBS: antiganglioside monosialotetrahexosylganglioside (GM1) and GD1a antibodies
  - Miller Fisher variant: GQ1b antibodies
- Nerve conduction studies

- ■ Nonessential for diagnosis but useful for GBS classification
- ■ May have value for prognostication
- ■ Can be normal early
- ■ Abnormalities most pronounced ~2 weeks after onset of weakness
- ■ Assess at least four motor nerves, three sensory nerves, F waves, and H reflexes
- ■ AIDP
  - ❏ Motor nerve conduction—decreased velocity
  - ❏ Distal motor latency—prolonged
  - ❏ F-wave latency—increased
  - ❏ Multifocal conduction blocks
  - ❏ Temporal dispersion of compound muscle action potentials (CMAPs) is abnormal
- ■ AMAN
  - ❏ Demyelination features are not present
  - ❏ Motor, sensory, or both have decreased amplitudes
  - ❏ Distal CMAP amplitude less than 80% of lower limit of normal in two or more nerves
  - ❏ If distal CMAP amplitude is less than 10% of lower limit of normal, you can typically find one demyelinating feature in one nerve
  - ❏ May have transient motor nerve conduction block
- ■ Imaging
  - ■ MRI of spine
    - ❏ Exclude high cervical lesion
      - • Particularly important if exam suggests a sensory level or if severe bladder/bowel dysfunction is present
- ■ Cultures
  - ■ Stool culture for *Campylobacter*
  - ■ *Mycoplasma* antibodies
  - ■ Viral polymerase chain reaction (PCR)/antibodies

ACUTE MANAGEMENT

- ■ Airway, breathing, circulation
  - ■ Airway
    - ❏ Assess ability to protect airway due to bulbar weakness or inability to clear secretions
    - ❏ Any disability to protect airway requires intubation
  - ■ Breathing
    - ❏ Low threshold for intubation

Fast Facts

There is *no role* for bilevel positive airway pressure (BIPAP) in patients with GBS because this is a progressive illness. Elective intubations are preferred over emergent because of hemodynamic instability that can occur as a result of concomitant autonomic instability.

- Progressive weakness may result in inability to take adequate respirations or even trigger the ventilator
  - Use mandatory ventilation modes
  - Ventilator should not be weaned until vital capacity is more than 1,000 mL
  - Patients with GBS often benefit from early tracheostomy to facilitate slow wean from the ventilator
    - It is important to explain to families that this can be removed and reversed over time; most patients require less than 1 month of mechanical ventilation

Fast Facts

Negative inspiratory force (NIF) and forced vital capacity (FVC) should be monitored serially. FVC less than 1 L or NIF weaker than –20 cm H_2O indicates the need for intubation.

- Circulation
  - Autonomic instability that occurs may require use of antihypertensive agents or vasopressors
  - Utilize medications with short half-lives
  - Be cautious to not "overtreat" hyper/hypotension, as swings can easily occur in the opposite direction and these patients often have increased sensitivity to medications

Fast Facts

Try utilizing alternative methods prior to medication for hemo-dynamic swings. Vital signs should be taken frequently and may change rapidly.

- Supportive care
  - Pain control
    - In addition to standard pain control therapies (acetaminophen, opioid narcotics), consider use of alternative agents such as gabapentin therapy or ketamine infusion
  - Fluid status
    - Ensure adequate volume status, as hypovolemia may worsen hemodynamic lability
    - Consider fluid bolus prior to initiation of vasopressors in hypotensive patients
  - Deep vein thrombosis (DVT) prevention
  - Nutrition

TREATMENT

- Immunotherapy with plasma exchange or intravenous immunoglobulin (IVIG) is the first-line therapy
  - Plasma exchange
    - Use within the first 2 weeks of onset
    - Typical course is five exchanges over 2 weeks
    - Use albumin as replacement fluid
  - IVIG
    - Start within the first 2 weeks of onset
    - Typical course is five doses over 5 days
  - Experimental therapy with eculizumab

Fast Facts

There is *no role* for steroids in GBS, as they are not effective.

PROGNOSIS

- Three to seven percent mortality rate
  - Death attributable to respiratory failure and complications or autonomic complications
- Twenty percent of patients remain significantly disabled at 6 months, 15% at 1 year
- Improvement can continue to occur after 3 or more years

- Most patients are able to walk unassisted by 3 months and have full recovery by 6 months
  - In severe cases, permanent disability can occur
- Persistent pain and fatigue are common in patients as a result of axonal loss
- Relapse can occur

Bibliography

Alshekhlee, A., Hussain, Z., Sultan, B., & Katirji, B. (2008). Guillain–Barré syndrome: Incidence and mortality rates in US hospitals. *Neurology, 70,* 1608–1613. doi:10.1212/01.wnl.0000310983.38724.d4

Hughes, R.A.C., Brassington, R., Gunn, A., & van Doorn, P.A. (2016). Corticosteroids for Guillain-Barré syndrome. *Cochrane Database of Systematic Reviews, 2016*(10), CD001446. doi:10.1002/14651858 .CD001446.pub5

Seneviratne, U. (2000). Guillain–Barré syndrome. *Postgraduate Medical Journal, 76,* 774–782. doi:10.1136/pgmj.76.902.774

11

Myasthenia Gravis

Myasthenia gravis (MG) is an autoimmune disorder of the neuromuscular system that causes weakness of the skeletal muscles. This typically can be treated on neurology floors or even outpatient settings. Myasthenic crisis, however, is a medical emergency and requires neurocritical care for management. Unless the diagnosis of MG has already been made, it can be challenging in the acute setting to diagnose and properly treat this disorder.

In this chapter, you will learn how to:

- Describe symptoms of MG.
- Diagnose MG.
- Review treatment strategies in both MG maintenance and myasthenic crisis.

EPIDEMIOLOGY

- Affects 20 in 100,000 persons
- Affects both men and women
- Affects all racial and ethnic groups
- Not believed to be inherited
  - Occasionally can occur in more than one member of the same family
  - Neonatal MG occurs when fetus acquires antibodies from mother with MG

- ❏ Temporary
- ❏ Symptoms abate 2 to 3 months after birth
- ■ Bimodal incidence
  - ■ Women peak during their 20s and 30s
  - ■ Men peak during their 70s and 80s

PATHOPHYSIOLOGY

MG is an autoimmune disorder caused by the disruption of acetylcholine traveling from the nerve ending and binding at the acetylcholine receptors due to the production of autoantibodies that block the acetylcholine receptors at the neuromuscular junction, thereby preventing muscle activation and contraction. In patients without MG, less acetylcholine is released into the neuromuscular junction with each impulse. In patients with MG, this presents as fatigable weakness, which is a hallmark finding of the disease.

Most commonly, this occurs as a result of antiacetylcholine receptor antibodies (anti-AChR Abs) that bind with acetylcholine receptors and not only block acetylcholine binding but also mark the complex for destruction. This can also occur as a result of generation of antibodies to other proteins, however, such as muscle-specific kinase (MuSK), which can also affect acetylcholine transmission at the neuromuscular junction.

The thymus is a gland responsible for immune function. The role of the thymus in MG is incompletely understood.

Fast Facts

Some scientists believe that in MG the thymus incorrectly codes developing T cells to produce acetylcholine receptor antibodies and attack its own cells, ultimately catalyzing the attack on neuromuscular transmission.

The thymus is typically largest in childhood, with its size peaking before puberty. It gradually gets smaller from puberty on, until it is replaced by fat. Throughout childhood, the thymus is responsible for the production of T lymphocytes. In adults with MG, the thymus remains large. It is common for patients with MG and a large thymus to have lymphoid hyperplasia, which does not usually occur unless there is an active immune response. In some individuals, it may develop tumors of the thymus (thymomas), which are often benign but can be malignant.

SIGNS AND SYMPTOMS

- Fatigable weakness, which improves with rest
- Symptoms often variable
- Symptoms can fluctuate dependent upon time of day
- In ocular MG (15% of patients), weakness is limited to extraocular movements and eyelids
- Facial muscle weakness is commonly the first observed symptom
  - Ptosis—drooping of eyelids (one or both)
    - Half of patients present with this feature
  - Diplopia—blurred or double vision
  - Change in facial expression
  - Dysphagia—difficulty swallowing
  - Dyspnea or shortness of breath
  - Dysarthria—impaired speech or trouble speaking
  - Weakness in extremities (necks, arms, hands, fingers, or legs)

Fast Facts

Pupillary response remains intact in MG patients and can help differentiate between other disease processes.

- Progressive weakness typically starts with ocular and progresses through the following groups: facial, bulbar, truncal, appendicular.
- Approximately one of five patients present in myasthenic crisis

DIAGNOSIS

- Thorough medical history
  - Weakness is a common symptom for many disorders, so diagnosis of MG is often delayed or missed until the time of crisis
  - High clinical suspicion if the patient describes weakness, which worsens with sustained activity but rapidly improves with brief rest
- Physical examination
  - Respiratory assessment, including measurement of vital capacity
- Thorough neurological examination, including assessment of the following
  - Eye movements
  - Coordination

- Sensation
- Muscle tone and strength
- Tensilon test
  - To perform this test, edrophonium chloride 2 mg is injected intravenously and muscle strength assessed after 30 seconds; the 2-mg dose may be repeated every 15 seconds to a maximum of 10 mg
    - Test should be completed with cardiac monitoring and atropine at bedside
  - An affirmative test demonstrates definitive improvement in muscle strength
  - Edrophonium blocks acetylcholine breakdown and increases levels of acetylcholine at the neuromuscular junction
- Ice-pack test
  - To perform this test, an ice pack is placed over the eyelids for several minutes
  - An affirmative test demonstrates improvement in ptosis by 2 mm or more
  - Reduced muscle temperature can inhibit acetylcholinesterase (AChE) activity
- Blood testing
  - Anti-AChR Abs should be checked first
    - Present or elevated
    - Levels do not correlate with severity of illness

Fast Facts

Only test for other antibodies if anti-AChR Ab is *not* present. It is the most specific and is present in over 80% of patients with MG.

- Anti-MuSK antibody
  - Present in half of MG patients who do not have anti-AChR Abs
- Less common antibodies
  - Anti-LRP4
  - Antiagrin
- Seronegative MG
  - Does not have either of the aforementioned antibodies
- Electromyography (EMG)
  - Stimulates nerves repeatedly to tire specific muscles; in MG, muscles do not respond as well as muscles in patients without the disorder
    - Affirmative test if greater than 10% decrease in nerve conduction study (NCS) with repetitive stimulation of a peripheral nerve at 2 to 5 Hz

- Single-fiber EMG
  - Detects impaired nerve-to-muscle transmission
  - Affirmative test if increased jitter
  - Most sensitive test for MG, but not specific
  - Sensitive in diagnosing mild cases that would go undetected by other testing modalities
- Imaging
  - Chest CT or MRI may identify presence of thymoma

Fast Facts

CT or MRI of brain is *not* indicated in the diagnosis of MG, though it is not uncommon to see these tests completed to rule out alternative causes for weakness.

TREATMENT

- MG can be treated but not cured
- May require ICU admission during times of crisis (Table 11.1)
- Anticholinesterase medications
  - Mestinon or pyridostigmine: slow acetylcholine breakdown at the neuromuscular junction that improves neuromuscular transmission and muscle strength
- Immunosuppressive drugs
  - Azathioprine, rituximab
  - Mycophenolate mofetil
  - Tacrolimus
  - Steroids, such as prednisone

Table 11.1

Widely Accepted Criteria for ICU Admission for MG
Vital capacity <20 mL/kg
NIF <20 cm H_2O
Weak neck flexors, drooling, inability to control oral secretions
Airway protection concern (bulbar weakness)
Need for mechanical ventilation
Pulmonary infiltrates
Need for plasma exchange monitoring

MG, myasthenia gravis; NIF, negative inspiratory force.

- Thymectomy
  - Operation that removes the thymus gland
  - Beneficial to patients with and without thymoma by reducing muscle weakness and need for immunosuppressive drugs
  - Fifty percent of patients achieve long-lasting remission
- Plasmapheresis
  - Removes antibodies from plasma and replaces with plasma or plasma substitute
  - Requires dialysis catheter
  - Temporarily effective
- Intravenous immunoglobulin (IVIG)
  - Concentrated injection of pooled antibodies from healthy donors
  - Binds with antibodies that cause MG and removes them from circulation
  - Temporarily changes immune system operation

MYASTHENIC CRISIS

- Medical emergency where muscles that control respiratory function have failed
- Fifteen to twenty percent of MG patients experience at least one myasthenic crisis
- The first myasthenic crisis commonly occurs within the first year following diagnosis
- Often occurs following trigger (Table 11.2)

Table 11.2

Common Myasthenic Crisis Triggers
Infection (most commonly seen following pulmonary infections)
Surgery (occurs following >30% of thymectomies)
Aspiration pneumonitis
Stress
Pregnancy
Extreme temperatures
Sleep deprivation
Immune-modulating therapy tapering
Medication effect
No obvious cause (up to 50% of cases)

Presenting Signs and Symptoms

Table 11.3

Common Signs of Impending Respiratory Failure	
Early Signs	**Late Signs**
Anxiety, restlessness	Paradoxical breathing
Diaphoresis	Hypoxia
Accessory muscle use	Hypercapnia
Tachypnea	Apnea
Tachycardia	Normalization of respiratory alkalosis
Weak neck flexion/extension	Decreased level of consciousness
Orthopnea	Gurgling with respiration
Staccato speech	—
Difficulty handling oral secretions	—
Weak cough/gag/jaw closure	—

Management of Respiratory Failure

- Early ICU admission for patients who meet the following criteria
  - Severe bulbar weakness
  - Early or late signs of neuromuscular respiratory failure (Table 11.3)
  - Any abnormal vital signs

Fast Facts

Negative inspiratory force (NIF) and forced vital capacity (FVC) should be monitored serially; however, they are less useful in MG than in GBS owing to the waxing–waning disease process. FVC less than 1 L or NIF weaker than −20 cm H_2O indicates the need for intubation.

- Airway, breathing, circulation
  - If patients are not adequately protecting their airway, they require intubation
  - The ventilator should be set in a full-support mode and not an assist mode

Avoid neuromuscular blockade during intubation.

- Bilevel positive airway pressure (BIPAP) can be considered if the patient is protecting his or her airway and does not have rapidly worsening symptoms or hemodynamic instability
  - Only beneficial if used early enough
  - Ensure the patient has control of secretions or this could quickly worsen the situation

Management of Crisis

- Remove triggers that may have catalyzed crisis
- Supportive care
- Medication therapy
  - High-dose steroids are first-line medication treatment in myasthenic crisis
    - Patients may worsen initially following steroid therapy
- Plasma exchange (PLEX) or IVIG
  - Described in the "Treatment" section earlier in this chapter
  - PLEX may work more rapidly in patients with crisis
  - If one therapy fails to demonstrate improvement, the other can be attempted
- Initiation of chronic treatments described above
  - Important to discuss with patient and family that these therapies do not work rapidly and can take months to years to be effective

Mortality

- No cure exists
- Relatively low mortality rate (<5%) in patients with myasthenic crisis
  - Mostly elderly

Bibliography

Deenen, J. C. W., Horlings, C. G. C., Verschuuren, J. J. G. M., Verbeek, A. L. M., van Engelen, B. G. M. (2015). The epidemiology of neuromuscular disorders: A comprehensive overview of the literature. *Journal of Neuromuscular Diseases, 2*, 73–85. doi:10.3233/JND-140045

Skeie, G. O., Apostolski, S., Evoli, A., Gilhus, N. E., Illa, I., Harms, L., . . .
Horge, H. W. (2010). Guidelines for treatment of autoimmune neuromuscular transmission disorders. *European Journal of Neurology, 17,*
893–902. doi:10.1111/j.1468-1331.2010.03019.x

Task Force of the Medical Scientific Advisory Board of the Myasthenia
Gravis Foundation of America, Jaretzki, A. III, Barohn, R. B., Ernstoff,
R. M., Kaminski, H. J., Keesey,J. C., Penn, A. S., & Sanders, D. B. (2000).
Myasthenia gravis: Recommendations for clinical research standards.
Neurology, 55, 16–23. doi:10.1212/WNL.55.1.16

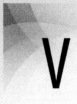

V

Seizures

12

Isolated Seizures

Seizures are commonplace and do not always require critical care intervention. However, it is also commonplace for neuro-critical care teams to be consulted for assistance in the workup of new-onset seizure. For the neurocritical care provider, it is essential to be able to recognize a seizure, determine when intervention is needed and the appropriate type, and know how to work up new-onset seizures.

In this chapter, you will learn how to:

- Define seizure.
- Describe seizure types.
- Detail workup of first seizure.
- Demonstrate measures to keep the patient safe during seizure.

DEFINITIONS

- Seizure: abnormal cortical neuronal electrical discharge(s) that typically cause a clinical event; symptoms are paroxysmal and vary dependent upon seizure type
- Epilepsy: two or more unprovoked epileptic seizures that occur greater than 24 hours apart
- Symptomatic seizure: caused by disorder of the central nervous system

- Acute symptomatic seizure: typically occurs within 1 week of acute neurological or metabolic disorder
- Remote symptomatic seizure: occurs longer than 1 week after neurological or metabolic disorder
- Provoked seizure: acute symptomatic seizure
- Unprovoked seizure: remove symptomatic or cryptogenic seizure (unknown cause)

EPIDEMIOLOGY

- Incidence
  - Single unprovoked seizure: 23 to 61 cases per 100,000 persons per year
  - Acute symptomatic seizure: 29 to 39 cases per 100,000 persons per year
- Gender
  - Unclear if gender differences are significant
- Age
  - Highest incidence of seizures in very old and very young
  - Incidence of age greater than 65 years is 100 to 170 cases per 100,000 persons per year

Fast Facts

U.S. emergency rooms see an average of 1 million visits for seizures annually.

SEIZURE TYPES

- Focal seizures
  - With awareness
    - Presentation varies dependent upon seizure foci (part of cortex from which the seizure originates from)
      - Occipital: flashing lights
      - Motor cortex: rhythmic movements of face, arm, or leg on contralateral side
      - Parietal: spatial perception distortion
      - Dominant frontal lobe: speech difficulties
    - Often precipitated by aura
    - May be followed by neurological worsening

- Todd's paralysis: postictal weakness
  - ○ Can last minutes to hours
- Impaired awareness
  - ❑ Presentation
    - Appears awake but cannot interact with others or his or her environment
    - May be motionless or have automatisms
      - ○ Automatisms: repetitive behaviors
        - – Chewing, lip smacking
    - May become aggressive
- Generalized seizures
  - Tonic–clonic
    - ❑ Presentation
      - Acute loss of consciousness followed by appearance of stiffening
        - ○ Apnea occurs and patient may become hypoxic and appear cyanotic
      - Following stiffening, muscles begin to jerk and twitch
        - ○ Patient may appear to be foaming at the mouth
        - ○ Tongue is often bitten
      - Postictal phase
        - ○ Slow, deep breathing
        - ○ Confusion or agitation may be present
        - ○ Patient gradually arouses

Fast Facts

Tachycardia and hypertension are common during seizures.

- Subtypes of generalized seizures
  - Absence
    - ❑ Childhood seizure
  - Atonic
    - ❑ Acute loss of muscle tone
    - ❑ Presents as collapsing
  - Clonic
    - ❑ Rhythmic jerking muscle contractions
    - ❑ Typically occur in upper hemisphere: face, arms
  - Myoclonic
    - ❑ No impaired consciousness

- Brief muscle contractions
  - Can occur anywhere but commonly legs
- Tonic
  - Acute muscle stiffening
  - Typically accompanied by impaired consciousness

INVESTIGATIONS

- Event description
  - Description of time leading to event
    - Triggering factors
    - Presence of aura
    - Progression
  - Event
    - Description of muscle activity and location
    - Length of time
  - Postictal period
    - Period of time until return to baseline
    - Clinical manifestations
      - Todd's paralysis
      - Behavioral symptoms

Fast Facts

Seizures have typically abrupt onset and progress rapidly, whereas migraine symptoms progress over 5 to 10 minutes.

Fast Facts

Most seizures end within 2 to 3 minutes. Prolonged symptoms have a wide differential diagnosis, including convulsive or nonconvulsive status epilepticus, migraine, transient ischemic attack, and psychogenic nonepileptic seizure.

- History
  - Prior events
  - Past medical history
  - Past surgical history
  - Family history

- Social history
- Medications
- Physical exam, including thorough neurological examination

Fast Facts

The presence of a lateral tongue bite has high specificity in distinguishing between psychogenic nonepileptic seizures and generalized seizures. In patients with partial seizures, laterality of tongue bite also typically indicates ipsilateral epileptic focus.

- Laboratory investigations (Table 12.1)
  - Glucose
  - Electrolytes: sodium, potassium, calcium, magnesium, phosphorus
  - Complete blood count
  - Blood urea nitrogen and creatinine
  - Liver function tests
  - Urinalysis
    - Pregnancy test, if indicated
  - Toxicology screens

Table 12.1

Differential Diagnoses to Consider When Evaluating Seizures

"SICK DRIFTER"

Substrates: sugar, oxygen

Isoniazid overdose

Cations: Na, Ca, Mg

Kids: Eclampsia

Drugs: cocaine, amphetamines, PCP

Rum: alcohol withdrawal

Illnesses: chronic seizure disorder, other chronic disorder, or acute illness

Fever: meningitis, encephalitis, abscess

Trauma: epidural, subdural, intracranial hemorrhage

Extra: toxicologic (TAIL: theophylline, aspirin, isoniazid, lithium) and 3 As (antihistamine, antidepressant overdoses, or anticonvulsant/benzodiazepine withdrawal)

Rat poison: organophosphate poisoning

PCP, phencyclidine.

Lactic acid and creatine kinase (CK) are typically elevated following seizure and do not necessarily need to be checked; however, they are valuable in distinguishing between generalized seizures and psychogenic nonepileptic seizures or syncope.

- ECG
  - May help to distinguish cardiac cause (Table 12.2, seizure mimics)
- Neuroimaging
  - All patients with first-time seizure without clear cause should receive neuroimaging to evaluate for structural abnormalities
    - MRI is best if not needed acutely
      - Can better identify mesial temporal sclerosis, infarcted tissue, tumors, or cortical dysplasia

Table 12.2

Conditions That Are at Times Mistaken as Seizures

Arrhythmias

Syncope

Migraine

Anxiety

Psychogenic nonepileptic seizure

Transient global amnesia

Narcolepsy (with cataplexy)

Paroxysmal movement disorders

Hypoglycemia

TIA

Dystonic reactions

Benign sleep myoclonus

Eclampsia

Rigors

TIA, transient ischemic attack.

Table 12.3

Orienting Novices to EEG Principles		
Left—Odd	**Midline**	**Right—Even**
F		Frontal lobe
T		Temporal lobe
C		Central lobe
P		Parietal
O		Occipital lobe
Z		Midline

Note: EEG is complex and cannot be mastered with one chart.

- ❑ CT if needed acutely, particularly if patient had focal findings or is slow to return to baseline
- ■ EEG (Table 12.3)
  - ▦ Acquire urgently if patient does not return to baseline
  - ▦ Otherwise, can be obtained routinely
- ■ Lumbar puncture (LP)
  - ▦ Not every patient requires LP
  - ▦ Obtain if concern for infectious process

Fast Facts

Seizures are often the presenting symptom in encephalitis. A high degree of suspicion for encephalitis should be maintained in patients presenting with seizure, fever, and normal neuroimaging.

TREATMENT

- ■ Medications
  - ▦ Most do not require medication administration
  - ▦ Benzodiazepines can be administered if seizure sustains greater than 2 minutes
    - ❑ Lorazepam 4 mg IV over 2 minutes
    - ❑ Diazepam 10 mg IV or rectal
    - ❑ Midazolam 10 mg IV or intramuscular injection (IM)

Table 12.4

Nursing Interventions During Acute Seizure

Before a Seizure If Aura Present

Priority is safety (have patient lie down)

Remove possible triggers

During a Seizure

Protect the patient from injury

Do *not* restrain the patient

Do *not* attempt to place an airway or tongue blade in the patient's mouth

Place the patient in lateral position as soon as the convulsion has stopped

Apply oxygen

Note details of seizure, including timing, level of consciousness, body part involved, type of motor activity, respirations, heart rate and rhythm, skin changes, pupil size changes, sensory changes, and behavioral changes

If seizure lasts >2 min, administer medication per provider order or call provider

After a Seizure

Perform neurological examination: note any residual deficits, including behavioral

Assess for injury

Review event for possible triggers

Note: These interventions could easily be performed by the advanced practice provider if present.

- Initiation of antiepileptic therapy is dependent upon underlying cause, risk of recurrent seizure, and patient stability
- Treat underlying cause
- Seizure precautions (Table 12.4)

PROGNOSIS

- Provoked seizure due to acute neurological insult unlikely to recur
- Unprovoked seizure has 30% to 50% chance of recurring over following 2 years (Table 12.5)
- Seizures resultant from metabolic causes do have risk of up to 3% chance of developing epilepsy
- Seizures resultant from neurological insults that cause permanent brain damage have 10% or greater chance of developing epilepsy

Table 12.5

Conditions Associated With Increased Risk of Seizure Recurrence

Age <16 or >65 y

Remote symptomatic seizure

Seizures during sleep

Previous provoked seizure

Previous febrile seizure

Family history of seizure

Status epilepticus or multiple seizures within 24 hr from initial seizure

Partial seizures

Todd's paralysis

Neurological deficit from birth

Developmental delay

Abnormal neurological examination in patients without remote symptomatic seizures

Brain tumor on CT scan

EEG shows epileptiform discharges

Bibliography

Farhidvash, F., Singh, P., Abou-Khalil, B., & Arain, A. (2009). Patients visiting the emergency room for seizures: Insurance status and clinic follow-up. *Seizure, 18*, 644–647. doi:10.1016/j.seizure.2009.08.001

13

Status Epilepticus

Status epilepticus is a commonly encountered neurological emergency that requires prompt recognition and treatment. Please read the previous chapter regarding seizures for initial management of a patient with seizures, as this is how status epilepticus starts. This chapter will go into more detail regarding diagnosis and treatment of ongoing status epilepticus and specifically into nonconvulsive status epilepticus (NCSE), which is typically much more difficult to recognize and manage.

In this chapter, you will learn how to:

- Define status epilepticus.
- List consequences of status epilepticus.
- Discuss the treatment algorithm for status epilepticus.

DEFINITIONS

- Status epilepticus: Two defining criteria are as follows:
  - Continuous clinical and/or electrographic seizure activity for 5 or more minutes, and
  - Recurrent seizure activity without a return to baseline between seizures
- Generalized convulsive status epilepticus (GCSE): Prolonged seizure with clinical symptoms, most commonly motor
- NCSE: Status epilepticus without clear motor symptoms
  - Diagnosis requires EEG and has specific criterion that must be met

Sustained eye deviation or nystagmus during acute altered mental status increases the likelihood that the patient may be in status epilepticus.

- Refractory status epilepticus: Status epilepticus unresponsive to first-line antiepileptic therapies

Convulsive seizures that persist for over 5 minutes are unlikely to stop and significant neuronal injury can occur.

EPIDEMIOLOGY

- Cases per 100,000 persons per year: 18 to 41
- Thirty-one to forty-three percent are refractory (two antiepileptic drugs [AEDs])
- Eight to thirty-seven percent of comatose patients in ICU
- Likely more common than one might expect, particularly in the following populations
  - Confused hospitalized elderly (16%)
  - Altered mental status (10%)
  - Traumatic brain injury (20%)
  - Stroke (6%)

CAUSES

- Low AED levels (Table 13.1)
- Stroke
- Traumatic brain injury
  - Subdural hematoma, epidural hematoma
- Congenital malformations
- Alcohol withdrawal
- Drugs/toxins
  - Cocaine, theophylline, isoniazid, tricyclic antidepressants, anticholinergics

Table 13.1

Dosing and Therapeutic Range for Common AEDs			
Medication	Loading Dose (mg/kg)	Therapeutic Range (mcg/mL)	Critical Result (mcg/mL)
Carbamazepine	—	4–12	20
Fosphenytoin	20	10–20	—
Lamotrigine	—	1–4	20
Phenobarbital	10–20	15–40	60
Phenytoin	20	10–20	40
Valproic acid	—	50–125	200

AEDs, antiepileptic drugs.

- Anoxic brain injury
- Electrolyte abnormalities
  - Hypoglycemia, hyper/hypocalcemia, hyper/hyponatremia, hypomagnesemia
- Hyperammonemia
- Infection
- Brain tumor
- Idiopathic
- Dieting or fasting
- Eclampsia

PATHOPHYSIOLOGIC EFFECTS OF STATUS EPILEPTICUS

- Neurological system
  - Neuronal injury
  - Secondary injury from other system effects (hypoperfusion, hypoxia, hyperthermia)
  - Intracranial hypertension
  - Increased cerebrospinal fluid (CSF) protein
  - Excessive intracellular calcium influx leading to cell damage/ cell death
- Pulmonary
  - Hypoxia
  - Respiratory acidosis
  - Neurogenic pulmonary edema
  - Aspiration pneumonia or pneumonitis

- Cardiovascular
  - Hypertension and/or hypotension
  - Arrhythmias
- Metabolic
  - Hyperglycemia and/or hypoglycemia
  - Hyperthermia
  - Lactic acidosis
- Other
  - Rhabdomyolysis, which can lead to renal failure
  - Leukocytosis

PRESENTATION

- GCSE
  - Easily recognizable
  - Physical manifestations of ongoing seizures
- NCSE
  - Stupor/coma
    - Generalized EEG seizure activity
  - Confusion with progression to stupor/coma
    - Focal NCSE, which then generalizes
  - GCSE that continues until motor movements stop despite ongoing seizure activity on EEG
    - Otherwise known as subtle status epilepticus

WORKUP

- History
  - Prior events
  - Past medical history
  - Past surgical history
  - Family history
  - Social history
  - Medications (Table 13.2)
- Physical exam, including thorough neurological examination
- Neuroimaging
  - Noncontrast CT of head
- Laboratory investigations
  - Glucose
  - Arterial blood gas
  - Lactic acid

Table 13.2

Common Medications That Lower the Seizure Threshold

Fluoroquinolones

Cefepime

L-Asparaginase

Cisplatin

Cyclosporine

Tacrolimus

Bevacizumab

- Electrolytes: sodium, potassium, calcium, magnesium, phosphorus
- Complete blood count
- Blood urea nitrogen and creatinine
- Liver function tests
- Ammonia
- Creatine kinase (CK), troponin
- Urinalysis
  - Pregnancy test, if indicated
- Toxicology screens
  - Urine drug screen
  - Ethanol (ETOH)
  - Therapeutic drug levels if on AEDs
  - Salicylates
- EEG

Fast Facts

Emergent EEG is indicated in patients with unexplained coma or altered mental status if a suspicion for seizures exists; these include patients with focal neurological deficits with no clear explanation, recent clinical seizure or status without return to baseline within 10 minutes, or clinical seizure that seems to cyclically start and stop.

- Lumbar puncture (LP)
  - In patients when there is concern for infectious cause

LP following prolonged seizures can sometimes have over 100 white blood cells (WBCs), which are not indicative of an infectious process and can thus cause confusion in interpretation and treatment.

TREATMENT

The goal of management is to prevent secondary brain injury and maintain adequate cerebral perfusion first and foremost and then to terminate the seizure.

- Medications (Table 13.3)
  - First-line therapy
    - Benzodiazepines

Early treatment is essential because benzodiazepines become less effective over time owing to changes in gamma-aminobutyric acid (GABA) subunits as seizure activity continues.

  - Second-line therapy
    - Levetiracetam (off label)
    - Valproic acid
    - Phenytoin
  - Third-line therapy (requires intubation and subsequent ventilator support)
    - Propofol
      - Bolus, followed by infusion
      - Works on GABA receptors, which decrease over time in status epilepticus, so may become *less* responsive over time
    - Midazolam infusion
    - Barbiturates
    - Clonazepam

Table 13.3

SE Emergency Medication Guide

Timeline	Medication	Dose	Route	Special Considerations	Rate
2–5 min	Lorazepam	0.1 mg/kg or 4 mg	IV	May repeat bolus	—
	Diazepam	0.2 mg/kg	IV	—	—
	Midazolam	0.02 mg/kg	IV	—	—
	Midazolam	10 mg	IM/IO/buccal	—	—
	Diazepam	20 mg	Rectal	—	—
5–10 min	Fosphenytoin	20 mg/kg	IV	*	Bolus rate: 100–150 mg PE/min
	Phenytoin	20 mg/kg	IV	*	Bolus rate: 25–50 mg/min
	Valproic acid	20–40 mg/kg	IV	*	Bolus rate: 5 mg/kg/min
First 60 min	Propofol	1–2 mg/kg bolus; infusion initial dose: 0.1 mg/kg/hr	IV	—	Maintenance range: 0.05–2.9 mg/kg/hr
	Midazolam	0.2 mg/kg bolus, repeat 0.2–0.4 mg/kg q5m; infusion initial dose: 0.1 mg/kg/hr	IV	May repeat bolus	Maintenance range: 0.05–2.9 mg/kg/hr
Super Refractory SE	Pentobarbital	5 mg/kg IV load; infusion initial dose: 1 mg/kg/hr	IV	May repeat bolus	Bolus rate: 50 mg/min; maintenance range: 0.5–10 mg/kg/hr

*Do not wait for antiepileptic medications to arrive; continue down algorithm, attempting to stop seizures. These medications, once they arrive, can be given concurrently with benzodiazepines or continuous infusions.

IM, intramuscular injection; IO, intraosseous infusion; IV, intravenous; PE, phenytoin equivalents; SE, status epilepticus.

Etomidate should be avoided during the intubation of a patient with status epilepticus, as it can actually activate seizure foci, and myoclonus is a well-known side effect. Instead, consider the combination use of propofol and ketamine, colloquially referred to as "ketofol," which has powerful antiepileptic properties as well as decreases hypotension risk.

- Fourth-line therapy
  - Ketamine infusion
    - Blocks *N*-Methyl-D-aspartate receptors (NMDARs)
    - NMDARs actually *increase* over time in status epilepticus, potentially improving the efficacy of ketamine over time
  - Magnesium
  - Thiopentone
  - Volatile anesthetic agent
- Other therapies
  - Deep brain stimulator
  - Ketogenic diet
  - Neurosurgical interventions
  - Hypothermia
  - Steroids

PROGNOSIS

- GCSE 30-day mortality rate ranges from 10% to 27%
- Mortality rate increases with prolonged seizures
  - Mortality rate if treated within 30 minutes is 36% but increases to 75% if treatment takes over 24 hours
  - Status epilepticus resolved in less than 10 hours has a 10% mortality rate compared to an 85% mortality rate when it takes over 20 hours to resolve

Bibliography

Brophy, G. M., Bell, R., Claassen, J., Alldredge, B., Bleck, T. P., Glauser, T., . . . Vespa, P. M.; Neurocritical Care Society Status Epilepticus Guideline Writing Committee. (2012). Guidelines for the evaluation and management of status epilepticus. *Neurocritical Care, 17*, 3–23. doi:10.1007/s12028-012-9695-z

Rossetti, A. O., & Lowenstein, D. H. (2011). Management of refractory status epilepticus in adults: Still more questions than answers. *The Lancet Neurology, 10*, 922–930. doi:10.1016/S1474-4422(11)70187-9

VI

Neuroinfectious Disorders

14

Meningitis

Meningitis is defined as inflammation of the meninges. There are many reasons that this may occur, and although the initial presentation may be similar, the treatment is very different dependent upon the cause. This chapter will help the reader identify meningitis as a differential diagnosis and discuss workup, cerebrospinal fluid (CSF) interpretation, and treatment.

In this chapter, you will learn how to:

- Recognize signs and symptoms of possible meningitis.
- Interpret CSF to confirm diagnosis.
- Discuss treatment strategies for different types of meningitis.

PRESENTATION

- Most common symptoms
  - Altered mental status
  - Fever
  - Meningismus (neck stiffness)
  - Headache

Fast Facts

In one study, less than half of patients had the once-called "classic" triad of altered mental status, neck stiffness, and fever, but almost all patients had at least two symptoms when headache was added.

- Additional common findings
  - Seizures
  - Vomiting
  - Cranial nerve palsies
  - Kernig's sign
    - Unable to straighten leg greater than 135 degrees without pain
  - Brudzinski's sign
    - Severe neck stiffness causes hips and knees to flex when neck is flexed
  - Jolt accentuation test
    - Can only be done with cooperative patients
    - Patient quickly moves head side to side in a horizontal plane; if headache worsens, then this is considered a positive finding
    - Positive jolt in combination with fever may be a more sensitive test than Kernig's or Brudzinski's sign.
  - Papilledema

Fast Facts

The sensitivity and specificity of Kernig's and Brudzinski's signs have not been adequately studied. Absence of these signs does not rule out meningitis.

- Atypical presentations
  - Elderly
    - Obtundation without fever or meningismus
  - Immunocompromised host
    - Altered mental status
    - No fever due to inability to mount inflammatory response

DIAGNOSIS

- Neuroimaging
  - Noncontrast CT
    - Do not delay antibiotic administration to obtain CT or lumbar puncture (LP)
    - Excludes alternative diagnosis, subarachnoid hemorrhage (SAH)
    - Evaluates mass effect
    - Obtain CT prior to LP in the following patients
      - Immunocompromised patients
      - History of central nervous system (CNS) disease
      - Altered mental status
      - Focal neurological deficits
      - Papilledema
      - New-onset seizure(s)
    - In some cases LP may be pursued *prior* to CT scan or without CT scan

Fast Facts

A high suspicion for meningitis should be maintained in patients with fever, headache, altered mental status, and a normal CT.

- LP
  - A diagnosis of meningitis cannot be made without an LP
  - Always obtain an opening pressure
  - Results will help to guide therapy
  - CSF testing (Table 14.1)
    - Ideally obtain CSF in all four tubes
    - The following tests should be ordered for all LPs
      - Red blood cell (RBC) count
      - White blood cell (WBC) count
      - Protein
      - Glucose
      - Gram stain
      - Culture
    - Consider these additional tests
      - Lactic acid (CSF)
      - India ink if suspicion for fungal infection
      - Herpes polymerase chain reaction (PCR)
      - Antigens

Table 14.1

CSF Interpretation

CSF Findings	Normal	Bacterial	Viral	Fungal	TB	SAH	GBS	MS
Appearance	Clear	Cloudy, turbid	Clear	Clear or cloudy	Opaque; forms fibrin web if left to settle	Sanguineous initially, xanthochromia >12 hr later	Clear or xanthochromia	Clear
Opening pressure	<20 cmH$_2$O	Elevated; >25 cmH$_2$O	Normal or elevated	Elevated	Elevated	Elevated	Normal or elevated	Normal
WBC count	<5 cells/µL	Elevated; >100 cells/µL; primarily PMNs (>90%)	Elevated; 50–1,000 cells/µL; primarily lymphocytes, can be PMNs early on	Elevated; 10–500 cells/µL	Elevated; 10–1,000 cells/µL; early PMNs then mononuclear cells	Elevated; WBC to RBC ratio of 1:1,000	Normal	0–20 cells/µL; primarily lymphocytes

Glucose	CSF glucose/ serum glucose ratio is >0.67	Low; <40% serum glucose	Normal; >60% of serum glucose; may be low in HSV	Low	Low	Normal	Normal	Normal
Protein	<50 mg/gL	Elevated; >50 mg/dL	Elevated; >50 mg/dL	Elevated	Elevated; 1–5 g/L	Elevated	Elevated; >5.5 g/L	Mildly elevated; 0.45–0.75 g/L
Causes	Normal	Adults: *Neisseria meningitides*, *Streptococcus pneumoniae*, *Listeria monocytogenes*	HSV (HSV 2 more common than HSV 1); enterovirus, varicella zoster virus, mumps, HIV, adenovirus	*Cryptococcus neoformans*, *Candida*	Tuberculosis	Trauma, vascular malformation	*Campylobacter jejuni*, CMV, EBV, *Mycoplasma pneumoniae*, varicella zoster virus	

CMV, cytomegalovirus; CSF, cerebrospinal fluid; EBV, Epstein–Barr virus; GBS, Guillain–Barré syndrome; HSV, herpes simplex virus; MS, multiple sclerosis; PMN, polymorphonuclear leukocyte; RBC, red blood cell; SAH, subarachnoid hemorrhage; TB, tuberculosis; WBC, white blood cell.

Patients with a normal CT scan are still at risk for herniation in cases of fulminant meningitis due to disease progression. This risk should be discussed at the time of procedure consent.

TREATMENT

- Treat every patient with suspicion for meningitis until ruled out
  - Administer antimicrobials immediately (Tables 14.2 & 14.3)
    - CT scan, LP, or blood cultures should not delay antibiotic administration
    - Any delay over an hour increases mortality rate by greater than 10%
  - Empiric dexamethasone if unclear source
    - Ideally given 10 to 20 minutes prior to or concurrently with first dose of antibiotics; do not give if patients have already received antibiotics
    - Dose: dexamethasone 10 mg IV × 1; then q6h for a duration of 2 to 4 days
    - Not necessary if organism is unlikely to be *Streptococcus pneumoniae*
  - Septic shock
    - Fluid bolus of 30 mL/kg IV over 1 hour
    - Goal mean arterial pressure (MAP) greater than 65 mmHg; the patient may require vasopressors to sustain after volume resuscitation
    - Trend lactic acid

TYPES OF MENINGITIS

- Bacterial
  - Epidemiology
    - In United States: approximately 3 cases per 100,000 people
    - Worldwide: ~500,000 cases per year
  - Treatment
    - Dependent upon organism
    - Initially broad coverage per Table 14.2

Table 14.2

Early Antibiotics Recommendations for Suspected Meningitis by Age		
Acute Symptom Onset (hours)	Age/Population	Gradual Symptom Onset (days)
Decadron + 3rd-generation cephalosporin + vancomycin	Young adults	Acyclovir
Decadron + 3rd-generation cephalosporin + vancomycin	Middle age	Acyclovir
Decadron + 3rd-generation cephalosporin + vancomycin + ampicillin	Elderly or immunocompromised	Acyclovir + Amphotericin B

Table 14.3

Suggested Antibiotic Dosing in Adults With Normal Renal Function			
Third-Generation Cephalosporin	Vancomycin	Ampicillin	Acyclovir
Ceftriaxone 2 g IV q12h	Vancomycin 15–20 mg/kg IV every 8–12 hr; not to exceed 2 g per dose or daily total of 60 mg/kg	Ampicillin 2 g IV q4h	Acyclovir 10 mg/kg IV q8h
	Trough goal: 15–20 mcg/mL		Based on ideal body weight

IV, intravenous.

- Prognosis
  - *Fatal* if not treated
  - High morbidity and mortality rates

Hospitalized patients should be placed on droplet precautions.

- Viral
  - Treatment
    - Primarily supportive
    - Patients with West Nile virus meningitis—high risk of respiratory failure
    - Discontinue antibiotics and steroids, if started for bacterial meningitis, once it has been ruled out
  - Prognosis
    - Most cases improve within 7 to 10 days
    - Some cases, such as West Nile, can take weeks to months
- Fungal
  - Epidemiology
    - *Cryptococcus* is one of most common causes of adult meningitis in Africa
    - *Histoplasma* in environments with bird or bat feces contamination, more common near Ohio and Mississippi rivers
    - Consider in immunocompromised patients
  - Treatment
    - Amphotericin B
    - Typically requires long courses of antifungals due to immunosuppressed state

Bibliography

Glimåker, M., Johansson, B., Grindborg, Ö., Bottai, M., Lindquist, L., & Sjölin, J. (2015). Adult bacterial meningitis: Earlier treatment and improved outcome following guideline revision promoting prompt lumbar puncture. *Clinical Infectious Diseases, 60*(8), 1162–1169. doi:10.1093/cid/civ011

Tunkel, A. R. (2001). *Bacterial meningitis*. Philadelphia, PA: Lippincott Williams & Wilkins.

Tunkel, A. R., Hartman, B. J., Kaplan, S. L., Kaufman, B. A., Roos, K. L., Scheld, W. M., & Whitley, R. J. (2004). Practice guidelines for the management of bacterial meningitis. *Clinical Infectious Diseases, 39*, 1267–1284. doi:10.1086/425368

15

Encephalitis

Encephalitis is defined as inflammation of the brain. It may present very similarly to meningitis. There are many reasons that encephalitis may occur, and although the initial presentation may be similar, the treatment is very different dependent upon the cause. Because there are different types of encephalitis, each will be covered separately.

In this chapter, you will learn how to:

■ Recognize signs and symptoms of possible encephalitis.
■ Interpret cerebrospinal fluid (CSF) to confirm diagnosis.
■ Carry out treatment strategies for different types of encephalitis.

PRESENTATION

■ Most common symptoms
  ▪ Altered mental status
  ▪ Motor and sensory deficits
  ▪ Seizures
  ▪ Cranial nerve palsies
  ▪ Suprareflexic deep tendon reflexes
  ▪ Hallucinations
  ▪ Memory disturbances
  ▪ Speech disturbances
  ▪ Hearing issues

DIAGNOSIS (TABLE 15.1)

Table 15.1

Criteria Required to Meet the Definition for the Diagnosis of Encephalitis

Major	Minor
Both criteria required	*Possible encephalitis = 2; probable/confirmed = 3+*
■ Altered mental status	■ Fever 38°C or more within 72 hr of presentation
Defined as any of the below	■ Seizures without an existing seizure disorder
■ Decreased or altered level of consciousness	■ New-onset focal neurological deficits
■ Lethargy	■ CSF WBC count ≥5/mm³
■ Personality change	■ New-onset or acute brain parenchyma abnormalities suggestive of encephalitis
and	■ EEG abnormalities consistent with encephalitis
■ Persists 24 hr or longer	*and*
	■ Exclusion of other causes of encephalopathy (trauma, metabolic, tumor, sepsis, alcohol abuse, others)

CSF, cerebrospinal fluid; WBC, white blood cell.

INVESTIGATIONS

- Laboratory evaluation (Table 15.2)
  - May be tailored based upon presentation or exposures
- Imaging
  - MRI
    - Most sensitive
    - Normal MRI does not exclude diagnosis
  - CT
    - If cannot obtain MRI
    - Obtain prior to lumbar puncture (LP) in patients with focal findings or signs of increased intracranial pressure (ICP)
  - Brain biopsy
    - Last resort for diagnosis
    - Rarely used

Table 15.2

Suggested Laboratory Investigations for Encephalitis				
Blood	**CSF**	**Serology**	**PCR**	**Autoimmune**
CBC	Cell count	Arboviruses	CSF	Anti-NMDAR
BUN/creatinine	Glucose	HIV	Throat swab	LG1
Electrolytes	Protein	Syphilis	Nasopharyngeal swab	CASPR2
C-reactive protein	Viral culture	Toxoplasmosis	Fecal	AMPA
Glucose	PCR: HSV, enterovirus, VZV, CMV	—	—	GABA-B
Liver function	Ziehl–Neelsen stain	—	—	Anti-Hu/Ma2
	Cryptococcal antigen	—	—	VGKC
	CSF IgG	—	—	GAD
	Cytology	—	—	DPPX

AMPA, α-amino-3-hydroxy-5-methyl-4-isoxazolepropionic acid; BUN, blood urea nitrogen; CASPR2, contactin associated protein 2; CBC, complete blood count; CMV, cytomegalovirus; CSF, cerebrospinal fluid; DPPX, dipeptidyl-peptidase-like protein 6; GABA-B, gamma-aminobutyric acid type B; GAD, glutamic acid decarboxylase; HSV, herpes simplex virus; IgG, immunoglobulin G; LG1, leucine-rich glioma-inactivated 1; NMDAR, N-methyl-D-aspartate receptor; PCR, polymerase chain reaction; VGKC, voltage gated potassium channel; VZV, varicella zoster virus.

VIRAL ENCEPHALITIS

- Herpes simplex encephalitis
  - Epidemiology
    - Most common infectious encephalitis
    - Five to ten percent of encephalitis cases
    - Most often occurs in people younger than 20 or older than 50 years
  - Specific features
    - In adults, typically caused by herpes simplex virus (HSV), type 1
    - Typically localizes to temporal and frontal lobes
  - Presentation
    - Flu-like symptoms

- Fever
- Malaise
- Headache
- Nausea and vomiting
- Seizures
- Behavioral changes
- Cognitive impairment
- Focal neurological deficits
- Diagnosis
  - Neuroimaging
    - MRI
      - Modality of choice
      - Abnormalities present in 90% of patients
        - Abnormalities are not specific to HSV
        - T1: hypointensities
        - T2: hyperintensities in the medial temporal lobes, inferior frontal lobes, and insula
        - Diffusion and fluid-attenuated inversion recovery (FLAIR) are more sensitive early
        - No changes within the basal ganglia typically

Fast Facts

Diagnosis can be challenging, as 5% to 10% of patients have a normal MRI and negative CSF initially. If there is suspicion, do not rule out HSV until another diagnosis has been confirmed or a second LP has negative CSF HSV polymerase chain reaction (PCR).

- LP
  - Raised lymphocyte count
  - May have red blood cells (RBCs) or xanthochromia if hemorrhagic encephalitis
  - Protein: mild elevation
  - Glucose: normal to mild decrease
  - HSV PCR
    - Early may be negative
    - Repeat in 3 to 7 days
    - Can remain positive up to 1 week after treatment
- EEG
  - Rules out nonconvulsive status epilepticus
  - Sensitive but not specific

- Treatment
  - Medication
    - Acyclovir 10 mg/kg IV q8h
    - Antibiotic course 14 to 21 days
    - Start at suspicion of infection
  - Supportive treatment
- Prognosis
  - Untreated
    - Greater than 70% mortality rate
    - Fatal in 7 to 14 days
  - Treated
    - Less than 20% mortality rate
    - Many survivors have neurological deficits
      - One half have severe deficits
      - One fourth have subsequent epilepsy

AUTOIMMUNE ENCEPHALITIS

- Acute disseminated encephalomyelitis (ADEM)
  - Epidemiology
    - Rarely diagnosed in adults
    - Most common in children under 10 years
    - Slightly more frequent in males than females
    - More commonly occurs in winter and spring
  - Special features
    - Often follows a bacterial or viral infection
    - Rarely follows vaccination
  - Presentation
    - Abrupt onset
    - Fever
    - Headache
    - Confusion
    - Seizures
    - Vomiting
  - Diagnosis
    - MRI
      - T2, FLAIR, and diffusion series
      - Multiple, bilateral, asymmetric widespread lesions
      - At junction of subcortical white matter and deep cortical gray matter
    - LP
      - Helps rule out other causes of encephalitis

- Immunoglobulin G (IgG) helps distinguish ADEM from multiple sclerosis (MS)
  - Brain biopsy
    - Rarely used/needed

Fast Facts

ADEM is diagnosed on brain biopsy when there is observation of perivenular demyelinating changes with axonal sparing.

- Treatment
  - High-dose steroids
  - Intravenous immunoglobulin (IVIG) and/or plasmapheresis considered when steroids fail
- Prognosis
  - Full recovery: 50% to 70%
  - Recovery can take up to 6 months
  - Mortality rate: 5% to 10%

PARANEOPLASTIC ENCEPHALITIS

- Epidemiology
  - Incidence largely unknown
- Presentation
  - Variable
  - Motor neuron dysfunction
    - Asymmetric proximal weakness
    - Neck weakness
  - Asymmetric facial numbness
  - Autonomic dysfunction
  - Paraneoplastic limbic encephalitis
    - Seizures
    - Sensory hallucinations
    - Sleep disturbances
    - Neuropsychiatric disturbances
    - Personality changes
    - Memory loss
  - Focal encephalitis
    - Seizures
    - Aphasia

- Weakness
- Numbness
- ▦ Brainstem encephalitis
  - One third of patients
  - Dysarthria
  - Dysphagia
  - Diplopia
  - Facial numbness
  - Hearing loss
- ■ Diagnosis
  - ▦ LP
    - Glutamic acid decarboxylase antibody (GAD Ab)
    - Cell count
    - Protein
    - Glucose
    - Oligoclonal bands
    - IgG synthesis rate
    - Cytology
  - ▦ Laboratory investigations
    - Carcinoembryonic antigen
    - Cancer antigen 125
    - Prostate-specific antigen
    - Complete blood cell count
    - Chemistries
    - Bleeding times
    - Liver function test
    - Vitamin B_{12}
  - ▦ Imaging
    - MRI
      - Typically unremarkable
      - May have T2 hyperintensities in mesial temporal lobes
    - CT/MRI of chest/abdomen/pelvis to look for malignancy
- ■ Treatment
  - ▦ Treatment of underlying malignancy
  - ▦ Plasmapheresis
  - ▦ No benefit noted from immunosuppressive therapy; still frequently used
    - Corticosteroids
    - Immunomodulators
      - Cyclophosphamide
    - IVIG

- Prognosis
  - Variable
  - Unknown
  - Some patients will proceed to coma and death

Bibliography

Venkatesan, A., Tunkel, A. R., Bloch, K. C., Lauring, A. S., Sejvar, J., Bitnun, A., . . . Glaser, C. A. (2013). Case definitions, diagnostic algorithms, and priorities in encephalitis: Consensus statement of the international encephalitis consortium. *Clinical Infectious Diseases, 57*(8), 1114–1128. doi:10.1093/cid/cit458

VII

Brain Death

16

Determination of Brain Death

There are two different ways to be declared legally dead in this country. The first is irreversible cessation of cardiopulmonary activity. The second is irreversible cessation of brain activity. Neurological examination findings in patients who have irreversible cessation of brain activity are clear. There are many considerations beyond just the determination, however. This chapter will describe brain death and its implications.

In this chapter, you will learn how to:

- Define brain death.
- Perform confirmatory testing for brain death.

DEFINITION OF BRAIN DEATH

The Uniform Determination of Death Act was adopted in 1981. This act provided the legal definition of death to include what is commonly known as cardiac death, which is the irreversible cessation of both cardiac and pulmonary function, and brain death, which is the irreversible cessation of brain function, including the brainstem. The act specifically does *not* give the criteria for the actual determination of death, other than state that accepted medical standards must be utilized.

There are essentially three components of brain death: coma from known cause, absent brainstem reflexes, and apnea.

WHO CAN PRONOUNCE BRAIN DEATH

- Laws vary by state
- Hospital policy may differ from state law
- Most organizations recognize that the attending physician can determine brain death if competent and experienced in the determination process
- Some organizations recommend a neurologist or neurosurgeon be involved in brain death determination

BRAIN DEATH EXAM

Typically in adults, only one physical examination is performed; however, some states, hospitals, or even physicians prefer to have two separate examinations.

- Known cause of coma
  - If unclear, further testing is needed
- Elimination of confounding factors (Table 16.1)
  - May require time to allow for drug or medication clearance
- Physical examination
  - Absent brain stem reflexes (Table 16.2)

Spinal cord reflexes can persist in brain death and are relatively common. This includes triple flexion to even sitting up with head movement toward one side. These are often referred to as Lazarus movements.

Table 16.1

Conditions That May Make the Diagnosis of Brain Death Difficult and Should Be Corrected and Controlled Prior to Formal Testing Being Initiated

Confounder	Rationale	Goal
Acidosis (severe)	Affects respiratory drive	pH 7.35–7.45; normalize baseline CO_2 as much as possible
Alcohol	Not always checked in trauma	Less than legal limit; <0.08%
Barbiturates	Long and sometimes unpredictable half-life	Level should be below therapeutic range
Electrolyte disturbances	Severe hypernatremia	Na <160 mEq/L
Hypotension	Can suppress patient's response to brain death exam	SBP >100 mmHg
Hypothermia	Prolongs drug metabolism	Core temperature >35°C
Medications (benzodiazepines, opioids)	Reversible, flumazenil and naloxone (Narcan) are not long acting so often will need to be repeated or given as continuous infusion	Remove from system
Poisoning, drug overdoses	Reversible	Clear toxins
Complicating medical conditions, such as hepatic encephalopathy, hyperammonemia, hyperosmolar state, and endocrine dysfunction	Reversible	Appropriate management of potentially confounding medical conditions

SBP, systolic blood pressure.

- Apnea exam
  - A study consistent with brain death demonstrates absence of respirations
  - Suggested test specifications
    - Ensure "normal" parameters prior to initiating exam
      - Core temperature greater than 36°C
      - Systolic blood pressure greater than 100 mmHg
      - $PaCO_2$ 35 to 45 mmHg
      - Euvolemia
      - No hypoxia

Table 16.2

Brain Death Examination and Findings	
Brainstem Reflex Tested	**Response**
Pupil	Absent; fixed and often dilated
Corneas	Absent
Oculocephalic	Fixed forward stare
Oculovestibular	Fixed forward stare
Facial movement to noxious stimuli	No response
Gag	Absent
Cough	Absent
Motor response to noxious stimuli	Absent

- Suggested method of performing exam
  - Adjust ventilator until eucapnia is achieved
  - Preoxygenate for 10+ minutes for a goal PaO_2 greater than 200 mmHg
  - Obtain baseline arterial blood gas (ABG) once SpO_2 greater than 95%
  - Disconnect patient from mechanical ventilation and place 100% oxygen via tubing to the level of the carina at 6 L/min
  - Observe for chest rise and fall or evidence of respirations for a period of 8 to 10 minutes
  - Obtain ABG

Fast Facts

Apnea testing should be aborted in the event of hemodynamic instability, SpO_2 <85%, or SBP <90 mmHg.

- Positive exam findings
  - $PaCO_2$ greater than 60 mmHg or rise of 20 mmHg or greater from baseline $PaCO_2$
    - Respiratory acidosis: pH less than 7.28
- Inconclusive findings
  - Test can be repeated for longer time period if the patient is hemodynamically stable

Table 16.3

Indications for Additional Testing in the Diagnosis of Brain Death
Inability to perform elements of the physical exam, such as in cervical or facial injuries
Inability to perform or complete apnea testing
Any inconclusive results
Family reassurance
Medical staff reassurance
Excessive spinal reflexes

- Limitations
  - Not valid in all patients
    - CO_2 retainers
    - Neuromuscular paralysis
    - High cervical spine injury

Fast Facts

If a patient "fails" an apnea test, this indicates that the patient initiated respirations during the exam. A patient who "passes" an apnea test is apneic.

Ancillary Testing (Table 16.3)

- EEG
  - A study consistent with brain death demonstrates the absence of electrical activity for 30+ minutes
    - Specifically demonstrates lack of reactivity to intense stimulation
  - Suggested testing specifications
    - Eight or more scalp electrodes
    - Sensitivity greater than 2 μV
    - High-frequency filter greater than 30 Hz
    - Low-frequency filter less than 1 Hz
  - Limitations
    - ICU devices may cause artifact that appears as false electrical activity
- Transcranial Doppler (TCD)

- A positive study demonstrates small systolic peaks in systole without diastolic flow
    - Otherwise known as reverberating flow
- Limitations
    - Some patients have poor insonation windows
- Cerebral angiogram
    - A positive test shows no intracerebral filling
        - Evaluate both anterior (carotid) and posterior (vertebral) entry into the skull
    - Suggested testing specifications
        - Patent external carotid circulation
        - Contrast medium is injected under high pressure
            - Seen reaching anterior and posterior circulation
        - Flow through the superior longitudinal sinus may be delayed
    - Limitations
        - Can be difficult to obtain if patient is hemodynamically unstable
        - May be presence of retained cerebral blood flow
- Nuclear medicine scan
    - An exam consistent with brain death demonstrates the absence of isotope uptake into the brain parenchyma and vasculature
    - Suggested testing specifications
        - Obtain images at multiple time points
    - Limitations
        - Difficult to obtain in hemodynamically unstable patient
        - Time consuming
        - May be presence of retained cerebral blood flow

Fast Facts

An image of the liver can be obtained to confirm isotope uptake.

- Somatosensory evoked potentials (SSEPs)
    - An exam consistent with brain death demonstrates absence of SSEPs rostral to N 13 and absence of P 14
        - Presence of N 13 establishes signal to the central nervous system
            - N 13 cervical potential, N 14 brainstem potential
        - Suggested testing specifications
            - Testing from nasopharyngeal electrodes may decrease false negatives/positives

- Limitations
  - Upper cervical cord and medulla lesions may show arrest of conduction with a present N 13 peak and absent N 14 and P 14 peaks
  - Should not be used if cause of brain death is brainstem pathology

Fast Facts

Evoked potentials may be useful in the evaluation of brain death in a patient who has received barbiturates during hospitalization.

Bibliography

Wijdicks, E. F. M., Varelas, P. N., Gronseth, G. S., & Greer, D. M. (2010). Evidence-based guideline update: Determining brain death in adults: Report of the Quality Standards Subcommittee of the American Academy of Neurology. *Neurology, 74,* 1911–1918. doi:10.1212/WNL.0b013e3181e242a8

17

Organ Donation

There are approximately 115,000 people awaiting lifesaving organ transplant. Despite widespread efforts to increase the donor pool, there remains a huge gap between those awaiting transplant and available organ donors. Hospitals are federally mandated to refer potential organ donors to their local organ procurement organization (OPO). It is the responsibility of the treatment team to preserve the option of organ donation for the patient and family even once the criteria for brain death is met.

In this chapter, you will learn how to:

- Identify appropriate referrals as potential organ donors.
- Describe the provider's role in the consent process.
- Utilize appropriate donor management strategies to optimize donor potential.

TYPES OF ORGAN DONORS

- Brain dead donors
  - Legally dead (declared brain dead)
  - Also called heart-beating donors
  - OPO manages patient
- Donation after cardiac death donors
  - Decision to remove support is made first and independently of decision to donate
  - Treatment team continues to manage patient

- Imminent death is predicted
  - Typically expected to die within 30 to 60 minutes after support devices are removed
- Recovery of organs for transplant occurs after patient's heart stops and death is pronounced

REFERRAL OF POTENTIAL ORGAN DONOR

- Identification of the potential donor
  - Call if the following criteria are met
    - The patient has a neurological injury
    - The patient has a Glasgow Coma Scale (GCS) score of 5 or less
    - The patient is requiring mechanical ventilation
- Other triggers to call
  - Discussion of end of life
  - Discussion of do not resuscitate (DNR) code status
  - Discussion of withdrawal of care
  - Discussion of brain death testing
  - Family brings up organ donation

Fast Facts

Early OPO involvement helps decrease the time family may have to wait while the patient is being evaluated for suitability.

CONSENT PROCESS

- Despite timely and appropriate referral, the family may not be approached for consent due to a variety of reasons (Table 17.1).

Table 17.1

Common Exclusion Criteria for Potential Organ Donors	
Deceased Donor (Brain Dead Donor)	**Donation After Cardiac Death**
Extracranial cancer within 5 y	Extracranial cancer within 5 y
Multisystem organ failure	HIV/AIDS
	Hepatitis C over the age of 50
	DCD over the age of 65

Note: These criteria are often set by the organ procurement organizations and may change dependent upon recommendations by transplant centers.
DCD, donation after cardiac death.

Ultimately, the determination of potential candidacy of a patient to be a donor is made by the OPO

- The consent process should always be initiated by the OPO or a designated requestor

Fast Facts

The mention of organ donation prior to this time is detrimental to consent success and is considered a "pre-approach." Organ donation should not be discussed by anyone other than the OPO or a designated requestor. If the family brings up organ donation, an appropriate response is "Let me find someone to discuss this with you" and the OPO should be notified.

- First-person consent
  - Patients registered on a donor registry or with an organ donor designation on their driver's license have consented to be an organ donor
  - The patient's next of kin is informed of the patient's decision, rather than asked for consent
    - The family cannot overturn the patient's decision to donate
- Formal consent
  - By designated requestor or OPO
  - Legal next of kin is approached
    - Timing
      - After pronouncement of brain death
      - After decision to withdraw care has been made

DONOR MANAGEMENT

- Goal: hemodynamic stability while evaluating organ suitability, finding potential matches, and procurement process
- There are eight organs that can be recovered for organ transplant at this time
  - Heart
  - Lungs (2)
  - Liver
  - Kidneys (2)
  - Pancreas
  - Intestines

- Promising research is investigating other possible transplant options
- Eyes and skin can also be recovered; however, it will not be discussed in this chapter

Organ Evaluation and Management

- Cardiac
  - Often require intravenous (IV) levothyroxine to improve hemodynamic stability
    - May be able to wean pressors once triiodothyronine (T_3) or thyroxine (T_4) is started
  - Evaluation
    - Echocardiogram
    - Electrocardiogram
    - May require cardiac catheterization if requested
- Pulmonary
  - Lung recruitment strategies
  - Aggressive chest physiotherapy and percussion
  - Empiric antibiotics
  - Evaluation
    - Arterial blood gases
    - Chest radiographs
    - May require bronchoscopy
- Volume status
  - Kidney and liver function might improve with volume resuscitation; however, this can negatively impact pulmonary function and/or cause the pancreas to become edematous—making it difficult to recover

Fast Facts

The Rule of 100s: In general, a patient with a temperature of 100°F, heart rate of 100 beats/minute, systolic blood pressure of 100 mmHg, oxygen saturation of 100%, and urine output of 100 mL/hr is considered to be in good shape.

Organ Recovery Process

- Once organs are evaluated, donor information is inputted into a database shared with transplant centers
- Organs are allocated to the sickest, closest patient first

- The transplant center can accept or reject
- If rejected, the organ continues to be offered down the transplant waiting list until accepted
- Operation time is set and organs are recovered
- Recovered organs are transported back to the transplant center
- Organ is transplanted

Fast Facts

Despite great strides in education regarding the organ donation process, misinformation is still prevalent and the topic can be controversial. For the families that choose to consent to organ donation, it is not uncommon for them to state that donation was the only good thing that could come from an otherwise bad situation.

Appendix A

N I H STROKE SCALE

Interval: [ ] Baseline   [ ] 2 hours post treatment   [ ] 24 hours post onset of symptoms ±20 minutes   [ ] 7-10 days   [ ] 3 months   [ ] Other_____ _____(__ __)

Time:____:____ [ ]am [ ]pm

Person Administering Scale _____

Administer stroke scale items in the order listed. Record performance in each category after each subscale exam. Do not go back and change scores. Follow directions provided for each exam technique. Scores should reflect what the patient does, not what the clinician thinks the patient can do. The clinician should record answers while administering the exam and work quickly. Except where indicated, the patient should not be coached (i.e., repeated requests to patient to make a special effort).

N I H
STROKE
SCALE

Patient Identification. ___-___-___

Pt. Date of Birth ___/___/___

Hospital _____ (___-___)

Date of Exam ___/___/___

Interval: [ ] Baseline   [ ] 2 hours post treatment   [ ] 24 hours post onset of symptoms ±20 minutes   [ ] 7-10 days   [ ] 3 months   [ ] Other _____ (___)

Instructions	Scale Definition	Score
1a. Level of Consciousness: The investigator must choose a response if a full evaluation is prevented by such obstacles as an endotracheal tube, language barrier, orotracheal trauma/bandages. A 3 is scored only if the patient makes no movement (other than reflexive posturing) in response to noxious stimulation.	0 = **Alert;** keenly responsive. 1 = **Not alert;** but arousable by minor stimulation to obey, answer, or respond. 2 = **Not alert;** requires repeated stimulation to attend, or is obtunded and requires strong or painful stimulation to make movements (not stereotyped). 3 = Responds only with reflex motor or autonomic effects or totally unresponsive, flaccid, and areflexic.	___
1b. LOC Questions: The patient is asked the month and his/her age. The answer must be correct - there is no partial credit for being close. Aphasic and stuporous patients who do not comprehend the questions will score 2. Patients unable to speak because of endotracheal intubation, orotracheal trauma, severe dysarthria from any cause, language barrier, or any other problem not secondary to aphasia are given a 1. It is important that only the initial answer be graded and that the examiner not "help" the patient with verbal or non-verbal cues.	0 = **Answers** both questions correctly. 1 = **Answers** one question correctly. 2 = **Answers** neither question correctly.	___

1c. LOC Commands: The patient is asked to open and close the eyes and then to grip and release the non-paretic hand. Substitute another one step command if the hands cannot be used. Credit is given if an unequivocal attempt is made but not completed due to weakness. If the patient does not respond to command, the task should be demonstrated to him or her (pantomime), and the result scored (i.e., follows none, one or two commands). Patients with trauma, amputation, or other physical impediments should be given suitable one-step commands. Only the first attempt is scored.	0 = **Performs** both tasks correctly. 1 = **Performs** one task correctly. 2 = **Performs** neither task correctly. —
2. Best Gaze: Only horizontal eye movements will be tested. Voluntary or reflexive (oculocephalic) eye movements will be scored, but caloric testing is not done. If the patient has a conjugate deviation of the eyes that can be overcome by voluntary or reflexive activity, the score will be 1. If a patient has an isolated peripheral nerve paresis (CN III, IV or VI), score a 1. Gaze is testable in all aphasic patients. Patients with ocular trauma, bandages, pre-existing blindness, or other disorder of visual acuity or fields should be tested with reflexive movements, and a choice made by the investigator. Establishing eye contact and then moving about the patient from side to side will occasionally clarify the presence of a partial gaze palsy.	0 = **Normal.** 1= **Partial gaze palsy;** gaze is abnormal in one or both eyes, but forced deviation or total gaze paresis is not present. 2= **Forced deviation,** or total gaze paresis not overcome by the oculocephalic maneuver. —
3. Visual: Visual fields (upper and lower quadrants) are tested by confrontation, using finger counting or visual threat, as appropriate. Patients may be encouraged, but if they look at the side of the moving fingers appropriately, this can be scored as normal. If there is unilateral blindness or enucleation, visual fields in the remaining eye are scored. Score 1 only if a clear-cut asymmetry, including quadrantanopia, is found. If patient is blind from any cause, score 3. Double simultaneous stimulation is performed at this point. If there is extinction, patient receives a 1, and the results are used to respond to item 11.	0 = **No visual loss.** 1 = **Partial hemianopia.** 2 = **Complete hemianopia.** 3 = **Bilateral hemianopia** (blind including cortical blindness). —

N I H
STROKE
SCALE

Patient Identification. ___ - ___ - ___

Pt. Date of Birth ___ / ___ / ___

Hospital _____ (___ - ___)

Date of Exam ___ / ___ / ___

Interval: [ ] Baseline   [ ] 2 hours post treatment   [ ] 24 hours post onset of symptoms ±20 minutes   [ ] 7-10 days   [ ] 3 months   [ ] Other ___

_____ (___)

Instructions	Scale Definition	Score
4. **Facial Palsy:** Ask – or use pantomime to encourage – the patient to show teeth or raise eyebrows and close eyes. Score symmetry of grimace in response to noxious stimuli in the poorly responsive or non-comprehending patient. If facial trauma/ bandages, orotracheal tube, tape or other physical barriers obscure the face, these should be removed to the extent possible.	0 = **Normal** symmetrical movements. 1 = **Minor paralysis** (flattened nasolabial fold, asymmetry on smiling). 2 = **Partial paralysis** (total or near-total paralysis of lower face). 3 = **Complete paralysis** of one or both sides (absence of facial movement in the upper and lower face).	___
5. **Motor Arm:** The limb is placed in the appropriate position: extend the arms (palms down) 90 degrees (if sitting) or 45 degrees (if supine). Drift is scored if the arm falls before 10 seconds. The aphasic patient is encouraged using urgency in the voice and pantomime, but not noxious stimulation. Each limb is tested in turn, beginning with the non-paretic arm. Only in the case of amputation or joint fusion at the shoulder, the examiner should record the score as untestable (UN), and clearly write the explanation for this choice.	0 = **No drift;** limb holds 90 (or 45) degrees for full 10 seconds. 1 = **Drift;** limb holds 90 (or 45) degrees, but drifts down before full 10 seconds; does not hit bed or other support. 2 = **Some effort against gravity;** limb cannot get to or maintain (if cued) 90 (or 45) degrees, drifts down to bed, but has some effort against gravity. 3 = **No effort against gravity;** limb falls. 4 = **No movement.** UN = **Amputation** or joint fusion, explain: _____ **5a. Left Arm** **5b. Right Arm**	___

6. **Motor Leg:** The limb is placed in the appropriate position: hold the leg at 30 degrees (always tested supine). Drift is scored if the leg falls before 5 seconds. The aphasic patient is encouraged using urgency in the voice and pantomime, but not noxious stimulation. Each limb is tested in turn, beginning with the non-paretic leg. Only in the case of amputation or joint fusion at the hip, the examiner should record the score as untestable (UN), and clearly write the explanation for this choice.	0 = **No drift;** leg holds 30-degree position for full 5 seconds. 1 = **Drift;** leg falls by the end of the 5-second period but does not hit bed. 2 = **Some effort against gravity;** leg falls to bed by 5 seconds, but has some effort against gravity. 3 = **No effort against gravity;** leg falls to bed immediately. 4 = **No movement.** UN = **Amputation** or joint fusion, explain: _____ **6a. Left Leg** **6b. Right Leg**	_____
7. **Limb Ataxia:** This item is aimed at finding evidence of a unilateral cerebellar lesion. Test with eyes open. In case of visual defect, ensure testing is done in intact visual field. The finger-nose-finger and heel-shin tests are performed on both sides, and ataxia is scored only if present out of proportion to weakness. Ataxia is absent in the patient who cannot understand or is paralyzed. Only in the case of amputation or joint fusion, the examiner should record the score as untestable (UN), and clearly write the explanation for this choice. In case of blindness, test by having the patient touch nose from extended arm position.	0 = **Absent.** 1 = **Present in one limb.** 2 = **Present in two limbs.** UN = **Amputation** or joint fusion, explain: _____	_____
8. **Sensory:** Sensation or grimace to pinprick when tested, or withdrawal from noxious stimulus in the obtunded or aphasic patient. Only sensory loss attributed to stroke is scored as abnormal and the examiner should test as many body areas (arms [not hands], legs, trunk, face) as needed to accurately check for hemisensory loss. A score of 2, "severe or total sensory loss," should only be given when a severe or total loss of sensation can be clearly demonstrated. Stuporous and aphasic patients will, therefore, probably score 1 or 0. The patient with brainstem stroke who has bilateral loss of sensation is scored 2. If the patient does not respond and is quadriplegic, score 2. Patients in a coma (item 1a=3) are automatically given a 2 on this item.	0 = **Normal;** no sensory loss. 1 = **Mild-to-moderate sensory loss;** patient feels pinprick is less sharp or is dull on the affected side; or there is a loss of superficial pain with pinprick, but patient is aware of being touched. 2 = **Severe to total sensory loss;** patient is not aware of being touched in the face, arm, and leg.	_____

N I H
STROKE
SCALE

Patient Identification. ___ - ___ - ___

Pt. Date of Birth ___/___/___

Hospital _____ (___ - ___)

Date of Exam ___/___/___

Interval: [ ] Baseline   [ ] 2 hours post treatment   [ ] 24 hours post onset of symptoms ±20 minutes   [ ] 7-10 days   [ ] 3 months   [ ] Other_____
(___)

Instructions	Scale Definition	Score
9. Best Language: A great deal of information about comprehension will be obtained during the preceding sections of the examination. For this scale item, the patient is asked to describe what is happening in the attached picture, to name the items on the attached naming sheet and to read from the attached list of sentences. Comprehension is judged from responses here, as well as to all of the commands in the preceding general neurological exam. If visual loss interferes with the tests, ask the patient to identify objects placed in the hand, repeat, and produce speech. The intubated patient should be asked to write. The patient in a coma (item 1a=3) will automatically score 3 on this item. The examiner must choose a score for the patient with stupor or limited cooperation, but a score of 3 should be used only if the patient is mute and follows no one-step commands.	0 = **No aphasia;** normal. 1 = **Mild-to-moderate aphasia;** some obvious loss of fluency or facility of comprehension, without significant limitation on ideas expressed or form of expression. Reduction of speech and/or comprehension, however, makes conversation about provided materials difficult or impossible. For example, in conversation about provided materials, examiner can identify picture or naming card content from patient's response. 2 = **Severe aphasia;** all communication is through fragmentary expression; great need for inference, questioning, and guessing by the listener. Range of information that can be exchanged is limited; listener carries burden of communication. Examiner cannot identify materials provided from patient response. 3 = **Mute, global aphasia;** no usable speech or auditory comprehension.	___

10. Dysarthria: If patient is thought to be normal, an adequate sample of speech must be obtained by asking patient to read or repeat words from the attached list. If the patient has severe aphasia, the clarity of articulation of spontaneous speech can be rated. Only if the patient is intubated or has other physical barriers to producing speech, the examiner should record the score as untestable (UN), and clearly write an explanation for this choice. Do not tell the patient why he or she is being tested.	0 = Normal. 1 = **Mild-to-moderate dysarthria;** patient slurs at least some words and, at worst, can be understood with some difficulty. 2 = **Severe dysarthria;** patient's speech is so slurred as to be unintelligible in the absence of or out of proportion to any dysphasia, or is mute/anarthric. UN = **Intubated** or other physical barrier, explain: _____ —
11. Extinction and Inattention (formerly Neglect): Sufficient information to identify neglect may be obtained during the prior testing. If the patient has a severe visual loss preventing visual double simultaneous stimulation, and the cutaneous stimuli are normal, the score is normal. If the patient has aphasia but does appear to attend to both sides, the score is normal. The presence of visual spatial neglect or anosagnosia may also be taken as evidence of abnormality. Since the abnormality is scored only if present, the item is never untestable.	0 = **No abnormality.** 1 = **Visual, tactile, auditory, spatial, or personal inattention** or extinction to bilateral simultaneous stimulation in one of the sensory modalities. 2 = **Profound hemi-inattention or extinction to more than one modality;** does not recognize own hand or orients to only one side of space. —

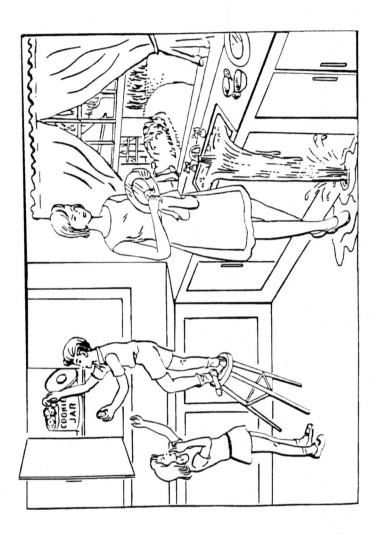

You know how.

Down to earth.

I got home from work.

Near the table in the dining room.

They heard him speak on the radio last night.

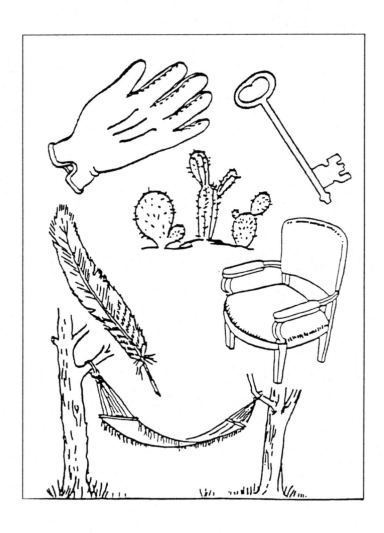

MAMA

TIP – TOP

FIFTY – FIFTY

THANKS

HUCKLEBERRY

BASEBALL PLAYER

Appendix B

INTERNATIONAL STANDARDS FOR NEUROLOGICAL CLASSIFICATION OF SPINAL CORD INJURY (ISNCSCI)

RIGHT

MOTOR KEY MUSCLES

SENSORY KEY SENSORY POINTS
Light Touch (LTR)   Pin Prick (PPR)

	C2
	C3
	C4
Elbow flexors **C5**	
Wrist extensors **C6**	
Elbow extensors **C7**	
Finger flexors **C8**	
Finger abductors (little finger) **T1**	

UER (Upper Extremity Right)

Comments (Non-key Muscle? Reason for NT? Pain?):

T2
T3
T4
T5
T6
T7
T8
T9
T10
T11
T12
L1

Hip flexors **L2**	
Knee extensors **L3**	
Ankle dorsiflexors **L4**	
Long toe extensors **L5**	
Ankle plantar flexors **S1**	

LER (Lower Extremity Right)

S2
S3

(VAC) Voluntary Anal Contraction (Yes/No)   S4-5

RIGHT TOTALS
(MAXIMUM)   (50)   (56)   (56)

MOTOR SUBSCORES

UER [ ] + UEL [ ] = **UEMS TOTAL** [ ]   LER [ ] + LEL [ ] = **LEMS TOTAL** [ ]
MAX (25)   (25)   (50)   MAX (25)   (25)   (50)

NEUROLOGICAL LEVELS Steps 1-5 for classification as on reverse		R	L	**3. NEUROLOGICAL LEVEL OF INJURY** (NLI)
1. SENSORY			
2. MOTOR			

This form may be copied freely but should not be altere

atient Name_____   Date/Time of Exam _____

xaminer Name _____   Signature _____

SENSORY
KEY SENSORY POINTS
Light Touch (LTL)   Pin Prick (PPL)

MOTOR
KEY MUSCLES

LEFT

C2
C3
C4

C5 *Elbow flexors*
C6 *Wrist extensors*   **UEL**
C7 *Elbow extensors*   **(Upper Extremity Left)**
C8 *Finger flexors*
T1 *Finger abductors (little finger)*

T2
T3
T4
T5
T6
T7
T8
T9
T10
T11
T12
L1

MOTOR
(SCORING ON REVERSE SIDE)

0 = total paralysis
1 = palpable or visible contraction
2 = active movement, gravity eliminated
3 = active movement, against gravity
4 = active movement, against some resistance
5 = active movement, against full resistance
5 = normal corrected for pain/disuse*
NT = not testable

SENSORY
(SCORING ON REVERSE SIDE)

0 = absent   *2 = normal*
1 = altered   *NT = not testable*

L2 *Hip flexors*
L3 *Knee extensors*   **LEL**
L4 *Ankle dorsiflexors*   **(Lower Extremity Left)**
L5 *Long toe extensors*
S1 *Ankle plantar flexors*

S2
S3
S4-5   **(DAP) Deep Anal Pressure** *(Yes/No)*

LEFT TOTALS

(56)   (56)   (50)   **(MAXIMUM)**

● **Key Sensory Points**

T2
C5
T1
C6
Palm
L1
L2
L3
L4
L5

SENSORY SUBSCORES

TR [   ] + **LTL** [   ] = **LT TOTAL** [   ]   **PPR** [   ] + **PPL** [   ] = **PP TOTAL** [   ]

MAX (56)   *(56)*   *(112)*   *MAX (56)*   *(56)*   *(112)*

4. COMPLETE OR INCOMPLETE?			R	L
complete = Any sensory or motor function in S4-5	*(In complete injuries only)* **ZONE OF PARTIAL PRESERVATION** *Most caudal level with any innervation*	**SENSORY**		
5. ASIA IMPAIRMENT SCALE (AIS)		**MOTOR**		

without permission from the American Spinal Injury Association.   REV 11/15

Muscle Function Grading

0 = total paralysis

1 = palpable or visible contraction

2 = active movement, full range of motion (ROM) with gravity eliminated

3 = active movement, full ROM against gravity

4 = active movement, full ROM against gravity and moderate resistance in a muscle specific position

5 = (normal) active movement, full ROM against gravity and full resistance in a functional muscle position expected from an otherwise unimpaired person

5* = (normal) active movement, full ROM against gravity and sufficient resistance to be considered normal if identified inhibiting factors (i.e. pain, disuse) were not present

NT = not testable (i.e. due to immobilization, severe pain such that the patient cannot be graded, amputation of limb, or contracture of > 50% of the normal ROM)

Sensory Grading

0 = Absent

1 = Altered, either decreased/impaired sensation or hypersensitivity

2 = Normal

NT = Not testable

When to Test Non-Key Muscles:

In a patient with an apparent AIS B classification, non-key muscle functions more than 3 levels below the motor level on each side should be tested to most accurately classify the injury (differentiate between AIS B and C).

Movement	Root level
Shoulder: Flexion, extension, abduction, adduction, internal and external rotation **Elbow:** Supination	C5
Elbow: Pronation **Wrist:** Flexion	C6
Finger: Flexion at proximal joint, extension. **Thumb:** Flexion, extension and abduction in plane of thumb	C7
Finger: Flexion at MCP joint **Thumb:** Opposition, adduction and abduction perpendicular to palm	C8
Finger: Abduction of the index finger	T1
Hip: Adduction	L2
Hip: External rotation	L3
Hip: Extension, abduction, internal rotation **Knee:** Flexion **Ankle:** Inversion and eversion **Toe:** MP and IP extension	L4
Hallux and Toe: DIP and PIP flexion and abduction	L5
Hallux: Adduction	S1

ASIA Impairment Scale (AIS)

A = Complete. No sensory or motor function is preserved in the sacral segments S4-5.

B = Sensory Incomplete. Sensory but not motor function is preserved below the neurological level and includes the sacral segments S4-5 (light touch or pin prick at S4-5 or deep anal pressure) AND no motor function is preserved more than three levels below the motor level on either side of the body.

C = Motor Incomplete. Motor function is preserved at the most caudal sacral segments for voluntary anal contraction (VAC) OR the patient meets the criteria for sensory incomplete status (sensory function preserved at the most caudal sacral segments (S4-S5) by LT, PP or DAP), and has some sparing of motor function more than three levels below the ipsilateral motor level on either side of the body.
(This includes key or non-key muscle functions to determine motor incomplete status.) For AIS C – less than half of key muscle functions below the single NLI have a muscle grade ≥ 3.

D = Motor Incomplete. Motor incomplete status as defined above, with at least half (half or more) of key muscle functions below the single NLI having a muscle grade ≥ 3.

E = Normal. If sensation and motor function as tested with the ISNCSCI are graded as normal in all segments, and the patient had prior deficits, then the AIS grade is E. Someone without an initial SCI does not receive an AIS grade.

Using ND: To document the sensory, motor and NLI levels, the ASIA Impairment Scale grade, and/or the zone of partial preservation (ZPP) when they are unable to be determined based on the examination results.

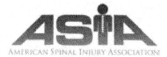

AMERICAN SPINAL INJURY ASSOCIATION

INTERNATIONAL STANDARDS FOR NEUROLOGICAL CLASSIFICATION OF SPINAL CORD INJURY

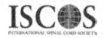

INTERNATIONAL SPINAL CORD SOCIETY

Steps in Classification

The following order is recommended for determining the classification of individuals with SCI.

1. Determine sensory levels for right and left sides.
The sensory level is the most caudal, intact dermatome for both pin prick and light touch sensation.

2. Determine motor levels for right and left sides.
Defined by the lowest key muscle function that has a grade of at least 3 (on supine testing), providing the key muscle functions represented by segments above that level are judged to be intact (graded as a 5).
Note: in regions where there is no myotome to test, the motor level is presumed to be the same as the sensory level, if testable motor function above that level is also normal.

3. Determine the neurological level of injury (NLI)
This refers to the most caudal segment of the cord with intact sensation and antigravity (3 or more) muscle function strength, provided that there is normal (intact) sensory and motor function rostrally respectively.
The NLI is the most cephalad of the sensory and motor levels determined in steps 1 and 2.

4. Determine whether the injury is Complete or Incomplete.
(i.e. absence or presence of sacral sparing)
*If voluntary anal contraction = **No** AND all S4-5 sensory scores = **0** AND deep anal pressure = **No**, then injury is **Complete**.*
*Otherwise, injury is **Incomplete**.*

5. Determine ASIA Impairment Scale (AIS) Grade:

Is injury <u>Complete?</u>   If YES, AIS=**A** and can record
ZPP (lowest dermatome or myotome
NO ↓   on each side with some preservation)

Is injury Motor <u>Complete?</u>   If YES, AIS=**B**

NO ↓   (No=voluntary anal contraction OR motor function
more than three levels below the motor level on a
given side, if the patient has sensory incomplete
classification)

Are <u>at least</u> half (half or more) of the key muscles below the
<u>neurological</u> level of injury graded 3 or better?

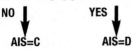

NO ↓   **YES** ↓
AIS=C   **AIS=D**

If sensation and motor function is normal in all segments, AIS=**E**
Note: AIS E is used in follow-up testing when an individual with a documented SCI has recovered normal function. If at initial testing no deficits are found, the individual is neurologically intact; the ASIA Impairment Scale does not apply.

Index